Hidden Secrets
of Super Perfect Health
at Any Age
Book II

Hidden Secrets of Super Perfect Health at Any Age
Book II

Twenty simple medically proven natural preventives and healing remedies to slow or reverse the aging process by many years

William L. Fischer

Fischer Publishing Corporation
Canfield, Ohio 44406

Hidden Secrets of Super Perfect Health at Any Age, Book II

Twenty simple medically proven natural preventives and healing remedies to slow or reverse the aging process by many years

Copyright © 1986 by William L. Fischer

All Rights Reserved

No part of this book may be copied or reproduced in any form without the written consent of the publishers

ISBN: 0-915421-05-4

Library of Congress Catalog Number: 85-080558

Printed in the United States of America

Dedication

This book is dedicated to the proposition that, for the most part, all people are created equally *healthy*. It's what we do (or don't do) for ourselves that makes the difference.

These pages are filled with stories of ordinary people who made some simple changes in their lifestyle and found their way back to vibrant health. I hope you, or someone you love, may have the same happy results others have had.

TABLE OF CONTENTS

Chapter 1
AN INTRODUCTION TO THE MIRACLES OF REBOUNDING 1
Rebounding For Boundless Benefits 2
   An Explanation of Rebounding 7
   The How & Why of Rebounding 9
   I Wanna Bounce! 18
   The Facts of Life 20
   The Decline & Fall of the Drugstore Rebounder 21

Chapter 2
SWEET, CRUNCHY, JUICY CARROTS
This Familiar Vegetable Offers Great Health Benefits 25
   Across The Ages 25
   Carrots Are Powerful Nutrition 26
   How to Enjoy Carrots 29

Chapter 3
VITAMIN P - THE NATURALIST'S VITAMIN
Together Forever: Vitamin P (The Bioflavonoids) & Vitamin C 31
   Vitamin P 32
   World-Wide Research 33
   Food Sources of Vitamin P 35
   Vitamin P as a Preventive 36

Chapter 4
TAKING A LOOK AT WHITE SUGAR
Is It Really A Major Health Hazard? 37
   All Sugars Are Not The Same 39
   Classic Symptoms of Sugar Toxicity 40
   Saccharine Disease 43
   NutraSweet 45
   Sugar vs Other Natural Sweeteners 46

A Special Word About Honey 47
What's The Answer? 49

Chapter 5
GRANDMOTHER WAS RIGHT ABOUT GARLIC 51
Folk Remedy Rediscovered 52
   Garlic Through the Ages & Around the World 54
   Scientific Studies Prove Garlic a Superior Natural Remedy 57
   Many Forms of Garlic on the Market 64

Chapter 6
THE MIRACLE OF LINSEED OIL
The Medicinal Fat 68
   Who is Dr. Johanna Budwig? 69
   Dr. Johanna Budwig Speaks 70
   Linseed - Past & Present 73
   World-Wide Research 76
   Some Heart-Warming Stories 80
   A Simple Suggestion 85

Chapter 7
MIGRAINE — ANOTHER NAME FOR PAIN
There Are Alternatives To Chemical Pain Relievers 87
   What Triggers a Migraine? 88
   Relief Without Drugs 90
   Tea & Sympathy 93

Chapter 8
VARICOSE VEINS
They're A Lot More Than Just Unsightly 94
   Cause & Effect 95
   Prevention Beats Treatment 98
   Summing It All Up 101

Chapter 9
THE NATURAL FOOD ALTERNATIVE TO CONSTIPATION 102

Constipation -
The All-Too Common Problem We'd Rather Not Talk About 103
    In Favor of Fiber 103
    Let's Talk Laxatives 112
    The Better Way 115
    The Antidote to Constipation 117
    The Natural Food Antidote for Constipation 122

Chapter 10
THE F-M CIRCULIZER SYSTEM
New to the U.S. — European Herbal Therapy 124
    The F-M System 124
    Circulatory Complications Are Many 126
    Empirical Evidence Abounds 126
    To Stimulate Circulation & Flush Away Toxins 130

Chapter 11
THE PROSTATE — WHAT IT IS & WHAT IT DOES ...132
UNDERSTANDING THE PROSTATE -
Everything You Need to Know About this Vital Male Organ .. 133
    Examining Prostate Disorders 134
    The Penis Prosthethis 139
    A Look at the Natural Preventives 140
    The Botanical Medicinals 143
    Additional Herbal Helps 146
    Massaging the Prostate 146
    Natural Biological Urges 147
    Conclusion 147

Chapter 12
NEW HELP & HOPE FOR THE IMPOTENT
Cause & Effect..148
    Identifying the Cause of the Problem.................148
    Nutrient & Hormone Deficiencies 149
    Drugs as a Contributing Factor 150
    High Blood Pressure 150

Impaired Circulation 154
Introducing Hanne Kramb 155

Chapter 13
Noel Johnson - 87 Year Old Marathon Runner
What's His Secret? BEE POLLEN 158
NOEL JOHNSON - The 87-Year Old Superman - A Profile 159
   Analyzing Noel's Secret Weapon - The Mighty Bee Pollen 166
   Examining the Evidence 167
   Choosing the Right Bee Pollen 170
   The Swiss Energy Formula 174

Chapter 14
SCANDINAVIAN DRY BRUSH MASSAGE 178
A Centuries Old Health & Beauty Secret 179
   The Skin is an Important Organ 179
   Defining the Problem..............................180
   Presenting the Solution...........................181

Chapter 15
THE CARE & FEEDING OF THE SKIN
Retarding The Natural Aging Process 185
   The Age Factor 185
   Characteristics of the Skin........................186
   Giving Nature a Helping Hand 188
   The Massage Oil 189

Chapter 16
FLUORIDE
Decay Preventive or a Preventable Danger?.............193
   Documented Fluoride Poisonings 194
   Not An Acceptable Risk 197
   The Cancer Connection 198
   Fluoridated Communities 199
   Escaping Fluoride Poisoning.......................201
   Spread the Word 203

Chapter 17
LITTLE-KNOW CANCER PREVENTIVES & SOME AVOIDABLE CARCINOGENS
Controversial Findings from Around the World...........204
- Laetrile - A Case in Point..............................205
- Dateline Europe 208
- Dietary Considerations 209
- Currently in Research 213
- Assisting Internal Defense Mechanisms 215
- At Increased Risk.....................................216
- Geopathogenic Zones 218
- Electrical Fields 219

Chapter 18
THE WORLD FAMOUS DR. RINSE FORMULA.........222
Jacobus Rinse, Ph. D. - The Man Himself................223
- In the Beginning 224
- The Dr. Rinse Formula - A Personal Account 227
- Nutrition for a Healthy Heart 230
- Dr. Rinse's Formula Praised by Many 240
- The Dr. Rinse Formula 246

Chapter 19
CONQUERING DEPRESSION & HANDLING STRESS
Nutrients & Support Therapies That Work 249
- Categorizing the Depressive State 249
- The Symptoms of Depression 250
- The Causes of Depression............................251
- SAD - Seasonal Affective Disorder 253
- Overcoming Depression Naturally 254
- A Concluding Thought 257

Chapter 20
CHRONIC INSOMNIA
Natural Aids for Healthy Sleep 258
- The Chemical Sleep-Inducers 259

Over-The-Counter Sleep Aids 260
Warning...261
The Natural Sleep Aids...............................262
"White" Noise...269
Practice Sleeping 270
Happy Dreams 270

Surprise Bonus
THE DR. STEICHEN SINK & STRUT
A Safe & Fun Little Exercise............................272
   The Steichen Sink & Strut........................273
   Dr. Steichen Says 275
   Aches & Pains 276

Epilogue
NOW IS THE TIME
Today is the First Day of the Rest of Your Life...........277
   What We Don't Know Can Hurt Us 277
   Take The First Step 278

Index 279

Disclaimer

This book is informational only and should not be considered as a substitute for consultation with a duly-licensed medical doctor. Any attempt to diagnose and treat an illness should come under the direction of a physician. The author is not himself a medical doctor and does not purport to offer medical advice, make diagnoses, prescribe remedies for specific medical conditions or substitute for medical consultation.

Neither the author nor the publisher has any interests, financial or otherwise, with any of the manufacturers, distributors, retailers or other providers of any of the products referred to herein.

While all case histories in this book are true, names have been changed or shortened to protect the identities of the persons described.

Foreword

I am pleased to add my voice to the praise being accorded *Hidden Secrets of Super-Perfect Health, Book II,* by William L. Fischer. I must confess that I became so interested in the diversity of material presented that I read the entire manuscript in one sitting. Because of my growing enthusiasm, I ignored my aching backside and need for sleep and continued reading through the very last fascinating page.

Hidden Secrets is well-researched, thoroughly documented, and estimably fair to the medical profession as a whole while presenting a strong case in favor of a preventive approach to the health problems facing the nation today. I myself strongly believe that, in many cases, the proverbial 'ounce of prevention' can beat a 'pound of cure.'

This book provides rare insight into the best of the old and new and offers a whole lot more than just an 'ounce' of prevention. It is certainly true that the task of the doctor will be eased considerably as more and more individuals learn the *Hidden Secrets of Super-Perfect Health* and put them into practice. It is 'required reading' for everyone everywhere interested in doing what they can for themselves to regain or maintain their good health. I recommend it highly.

Tom McCabe, D.Ph.

Preface

Hidden Secrets of Super-Perfect Health-Book II

By: William L. Fischer

Dear Friends:

Are you the type of person who sits down and makes a detailed list of 'things to do' - and then feels that the job is done? Are you the type of person who reads a 'how to' book - and then experiences a feeling of accomplishment without lifting a finger to practice what you've learned? Are you the type of person who buys a dress pattern and fabric (or some nails and wood for a bookshelf) - and then lets the material gather dust waiting for 'someday' when you'll finally get around to the project? If you are this type of person, you might as well pitch this book out the window right now!

I have been reading your letters for a long time now. What you tell me is that you want to know how to take a more active part in keeping or regaining your robust good health. I experienced a strong feeling of urgency while working with the material for this book. I hope that feeling of urgency is passed on to you as you read through the important health care information to be found within these pages. *Why?* Because I can do the necessary research and fashion the descriptive phrases and outline the preventive medicines and describe the healing therapies, *but only you can put them to work for you.*

Just reading about them doesn't get the job done. Wake up, America! Far too many of us are comfortable with our indulgences. In this land of plentiful fresh fruits and vegetables, we prefer to gorge on empty-calorie junk foods. We eat what we like, whether it nourishes our bodies or not. Many of us suffer from an unrecognized form of malnutrition that keeps us teetering on the edge of a real illness - or pushes us over the brink. We're too tired to care that we're tired all the time. We don't get enough healthy exercise to stimulate the flow of vital oxygenated blood and lymph through the circulatory system of the body.

I personally believe in effective preventive medicines and natural alternative treatments and therapies. I have seen the most astounding cures accomplished through basic changes in dietary and lifestyle practices. It is simply incredible what the human body can accomplish when it works with in conjunction *with* nature instead of fighting it. This book includes inspiring stories of many who have recovered their health by using the methods described in the following pages - in some cases, in spite of having been given a discouraging prognosis by the othodox medical establishment.

No matter how well researched, no book ever printed can take the place of a good and caring health-care specialist. This book doesn't pretend to be the one exception to this rule. Nevertheless, I have consulted with authorities around the world in order to bring you some tried and true time-honored remedies from the past, as well as some new and startling therapies and preventives that science is just beginning to recognize. If just one chapter makes a difference in the quality of your life and health, I will be well satisfied indeed.

William L. Fischer
Canfield, Ohio 44406

An Introduction to the Miracles of
Rebounding

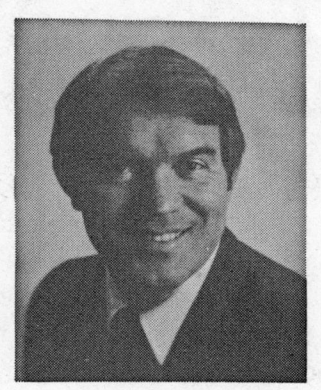

Al Carter has qualified twice for Olympic Competition. He has won 44 Gold Medals and 6 Silver Medals in amateur competition as All-Around Gymnastic Champion of five different states. He has won three state wrestling championships. Al Carter doesn't jog and he has never lifted weights—yet he can do over 100 one-arm pushups without stopping!

Al Carter is the designer of The Rebound mini-trampoline unit, founder of Rebound Dynamics, and developer of the Rebound Exercise program which has brought new life and hope to countless devotees of rebounding world-wide. Rebounding is unique among exercises in that it can be both gentle and simple enough for a wheelchair patient and yet so challenging and strenuous an Olympic athlete might select it as a training aid. But the real beauty of rebounding is that individuals of any age and in any state of health can benefit!

CHAPTER 1

Rebounding For Boundless Benefits

LAVERNE GROFF: HER STORY—"And they were married and lived happily ever after." Some fairy tales end that way, but the first seven years of my married life were a nightmare. I was in and out of hospitals more times than I like to remember. Less than a year after we were married, my husband rushed me to the hospital. My ovary had ruptured, I was bleeding internally, and the doctor said I was lucky to be alive. He had to remove half the ovary. Less than a year later, the same thing happened and I was back in the hospital for the removal of the other half of the same ovary.

A short nine months later, my other ovary ruptured and I was back in the hospital for my third operation. Each time I was admitted, bigger tumors and cysts appeared.

In the recovery room, after my third operation, my heart stopped. The quick action of the doctors and nurses started it beating again. A week later, after various tests, the doctors told me they found something else that had to be corrected.

After all these operations and so much convalescence time, I was unable to exercise. A short time after my last operation, my body just gave up. My nerves and muscles no longer functioned. I practically became a vegetable and couldn't talk for over two months. Someone had to feed me. I didn't have the strength to lift my arms and walking was impossible. My back was so weak I was always in pain. I began seeing a chiropractor and he really helped me. But as I began to learn to walk all over again, I was in constant pain from my back and my operations.

I prayed desperately, "Oh Lord. Isn't there any hope for me?"

Shortly thereafter, my husband and I were introduced to rebound exercise while attending one of Dr. Corwin West's self-help clinics. Dr. West told me he had seen only one other person in worse physical condition in his many years of practice. But we took home a rebounder and determined to follow Dr. West's instructions.

At first I had to sit on the rebounder with my feet on the mat while my husband bounced. We did this for a few minutes several times each day. In a few weeks, I tried it myself, sitting at first, then finally standing alone. As the months went by, I could feel my strength coming back. It was almost like climbing out of a dark grave into a meadow full of flowers. I was alive! My pain was disappearing. Not only were my arms and legs getting stronger, I could actually feel my insides getting stronger! Neither my family doctor nor my chiropractor could believe I was the same person!

After using the rebounder for a year, we wouldn't give it up for the world. We also have the most wonderful news that could have ever happened to us. We are expecting our first baby! The doctor said if I hadn't developed so much strength in my insides, I could never be carrying this baby. Considering the fact that we did it with only half an ovary, we thank our dear Lord each day for leading us to rebounding and Dr. West.

I want everyone to know this rebounder is the best thing I have ever found for eliminating pain without pills. I am now up to 15 minutes of running and jumping on the rebounder several times a day and I feel just wonderful!

NOTE: LaVerne Groff gave birth to a six-pound baby a few months after writing her story for us. Because of her previous health problems, her doctors were on the lookout for

4 / Hidden Secrets of Super-Perfect Health

complications. Instead, after keeping the baby in the hospital for five weeks as a precaution, they found the baby perfectly healthy and normal. Both mother and baby are happy and healthy and *home!*. Needless to say, dad is just as proud as a peacock!

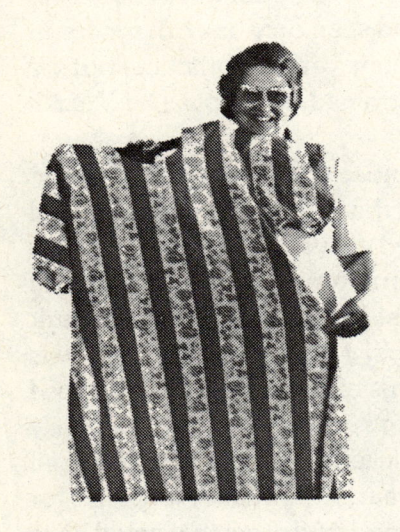

Dorothy Ross: "After just 2 ½ months, my backaches were gone. I had no more headaches, arthritis or bursitis pain and I went from a size 24 ½ to an 18½!"

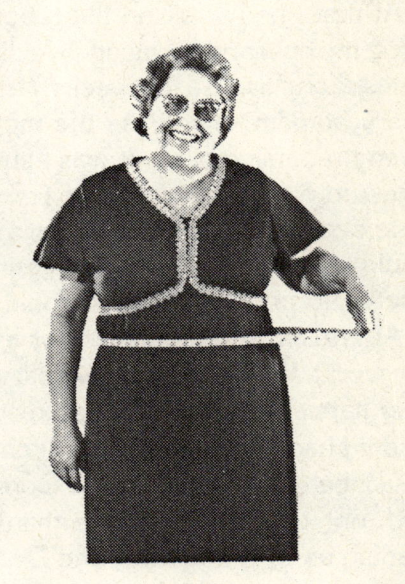

WALT & DOROTHY ROSS: THEIR STORY—My name is Dorothy Ross and I'm not going to tell you how old I am, but I'm the proud grandmother of 21 beautiful grandbabies... and I feel as good right now as I did when I was 35, but that wasn't true last February or the hard years before.

Early in the 1960s, I was hospitalized for a pinched nerve. The x-rays showed early arthritis had settled in my spine. My arthritis spread to my right knee and both ankles. I had bursitis in the right shoulder and both hips. I suffered with a constant backache and always felt completely exhausted. Other problems plagued me, too. The years seemed long with headaches, high-blood pressure, ringing in my ears, and poor balance. I literally cried many nights with pain from my bursitis. Walt finally bought me a four-inch foam pad to cover the mattress, but the pain was still excruciating.

Mind you, all of this had been going on for years on end and I was constantly under a doctor's care. He told me I was "just getting old and had to expect this sort of thing," but I didn't want to agree with him.

Walt had severe and painful problems, too. He suffered a heart attack, was found to be a diabetic a few years ago and had *four* cancer surgeries last year—two of them within 28 days! I worried about Walt and he worried about me. We were both discouraged and sick and tired of being sick and tired. We began to pray together for some form of exercise or *something* that would help us overcome our physical problems so we could enjoy life again.

After a week of fervent prayer, Walt brought home a rebounder. He was excited, but I was skeptical. For three days I watched him bounce for thirty seconds at a time. Each day he seemed brighter and had more energy. His disposition turned happy and sunny and he literally began to whistle while he worked, something I hadn't heard for a long, long time. I was just about ready to decide "it was all in his mind." I couldn't believe a simple exercise like bouncing could make such a change in any length of time, let alone just three days.

With his example, I tried to use the rebounder, but couldn't keep my balance. Walt held my hands to steady me and for three days, morning and evening, I did 25 counts of gentle bounce. Sure enough—I began to feel better, too! In two weeks, my blood pressure dropped 30 points, I had stamina, I lost 8 pounds and began to sing while I worked—literally sing! Life took on a whole new outlook. I had hurt for so long and been tired for so long, I had actually forgotten how it felt to feel really good—no, really *great*!

After just 1½ months, my backaches were gone. I had no more

headaches, arthiritis or bursitis pain. The leg and foot cramps that woke me up every night disappeared. I lost 20 pounds (!) and went from a size 24½ to an 18½. I heal more quickly and sleep soundly for the first time in years! No wonder I feel as good as I did when I was 35!

And listen to what rebounding has done for Walt! His stamina and recuperative powers have reached phenomenal dimensions. He lost 18 pounds and within a short period of time, could run a mile. His cholesterol level, which had always been too high and was the cause of his heart attack, is 10 points below normal. His heart-rate dropped 8 beats per minute and is now slow and steady. His eyesight has cleared. He now drives and watches television without glasses. The doctor says Walt is now in better physical condition than any time since he has known him and he might even be completely free of diabetes within a few months!

Are we thrilled and excited and happy to share the unbelievable benefits of the rebounder? You bet! Our whole life has changed for the better. We are happier, healthier, busier and eager for each new day.

Both of Walt's doctors were so impressed with his rapid recovery and incredible physical progress with the rebounder, it took only 15 seconds for each of them to decide they needed one themselves!

IN THE WORDS OF HARRIS NELSON: Harris Nelson of Hollywood, California—70 years young—sums up the benefits of rebounding in inimitable style.

"All you have to do is bounce on the rebounder, very easily at first (convalescents can sit on it), and it's astounding how it massages every organ in the body. The results have been fantastic! The concept is new. Bouncing puts all the cells in the body under stress. In defense, they fortify themselves, strengthening their walls. They become stronger and *so do you*! It's as simple as that! And it works!

"I need only six hours of sleep at night now—and no tossing as before—I wake up refreshed. No more getting up nights. Stress and anxiety reduced 100%. Cough gone. Arthritis gone. I can eat anything now, even before going to bed, and I don't wake up dizzy and nauseated at four in the morning because of my heart problem. NO ANGINA PAINS! I never enjoyed better regularity or elimination—it's perfect. I have renewed zip and vitality. I've lost eight pounds and no dieting. All muscles are firmer. My "pot belly" is reduced 1½ inches. I can read music faster. My mind reacts quicker—and I'm sure it corrected disorders I wasn't even aware of. Plus, plus, plus!

"All this—and why? Better circulation. Stronger lung power and a stimulated lymphatic system (your toxic poison and waste removal system)—action and movement. Exercise! And, happy day, I can do it all while watching television. No special garb, no sweat!

"And it's done all this for me in less than four months, exercising just five minutes twice a day. That's all you need to keep fit!"

An Explanation Of Rebounding

Just what is a rebounder anyway? Basically, the rebounder is mini-trampoline sized for personal indoor use. A circular unit of varying size, it stands 12" off the floor and the plasticized mat is suspended on a series of sturdy springs around its circumference.

In 1979, Albert E. Carter of *Gymnastics Fantastics*, the trampolining family which tours the country putting on incredible exhibitions of trampolining, published a book called "The Miracles of Rebound Exercise." Al himself attended Oklahoma State University on full scholarship for his wrestling prowess and has qualified twice for Olympic Competion. He was also All-Around Gymnastic Champion of five different states and earned 44 Gold Medals and

6 Silver Medals in amateur competition before turning professional 18 years ago. Pretty impressive credentials.

Al Carter, as a professional trampolinist, has been personally involved with rebound exercise for over 30 years. He is an author, a lecturer, and is considered a physical fitness expert. Al is the world's foremost authority on trampolining—rebound exercise—called the "most efficient, effective form of exercise yet devised by man."

When Al was first introduced by a friend to the household rebounder, he admits to being skeptical. (After all, Al Carter is used to highly professional and costly trampolining equipment, much too large for a living room.) Al remembers wondering how in the world anyone could jump on a trampoline in the average house without either denting the ceiling with his skull or hitting the floor through the mat, probably both. But he was impressed with the quality of the mini-trampoline and his words explain it best:

"It stood less than a foot off the ground on six round chrome legs and looked as if it were trying to hide by blending in with all the other furniture. I went over and picked it up, turned it over and attacked its soft underbelly fully expecting to find a fatal flaw. Surprisingly, I was impressed with the solid, quality construction. I carefully studied the stitching; it was strong. And I had to admit the springs were uniquely triangulated and of better quality than those on my professional trampoline. Each spring protected the other by not allowing its neighboring spring to extend to maximum length. I turned the unit over, set it on its sturdy chrome legs, stood back and looked at its profile.

"Ah-ha," I thought, There's the flaw. It's too low. No adult could bounce on that without hitting the floor. In fact, the fabric would probably rip out with any amount of use at all. I took off my shoes and stepped in the middle. It was surprisingly resilient. After a couple of quick, easy bounces, I put my heels together and thrust into the mat. My attack was met by an equal and opposing force that catapulted me into the air—and I didn't hit the floor.

"I felt a curious rising anticipation. It was as if someone had read my mind and developed this machine according to my specifications. This was possibly the first individualized rebound machine to meet my rigid requirements."

In a word, Al was "sold" on the unit and has become its strongest advocate.

Mind you, we have always believed the best way to find out about something is to go straight to the source. Albert E. Carter is unquestionably THE source for information on rebounding and its boundless benefits. We are indebted to Al for all the material on rebounding in this chapter, most of which has come straight from his book. After we prepared this necessarily brief "condensation," it was submitted to Al for editing and updating. Because we know many of you will recognize rebounding just might be the answer to your prayers, as it has been for so many others, we list Al Carter's address at the close of this chapter so you can go straight to the source for the name of a Rebound distributor in your area—and to purchase Al's book, "The Miracle of Rebound Exercise," the in-depth explanation of rebounding, known as the "bible" to enthusiastic rebounders every where.

The How & Why Of Rebounding

The common denominator of all forms of exercise is opposition to the gravitational pull of the earth. Think about it. Every exercise ever devised depends on gravity to make it effective. Push-ups, chin-ups, sit-ups, leg-lifts, weight-lifting—all depend on opposing the force of gravity with a specific part of the body. The aerobic exercises, such as walking, jogging or running, and the currently popular "jazzercise" classes, depend on the gravitational pull of the earth to be effective. Even in swimming, it is gravity that makes the water dense enough to create resistance to the musculature of the swimmer.

Gravity is the most important and constant physical force of our existence. You have to have opposition to develop strength. Where there is no opposition, there is no strength. To use the law of gravity for strength, we must oppose it.

Gravity, of course, is so much a part of our lives we don't think much about it. In addition, two other forces govern the way we get around—acceleration and deceleration. Gravity is a constant factor, but we can control acceleration and deceleration and harness them for our betterment. With the rebounder, we line up acceleration and deceleration with gravity. This is the purpose of the rebounder.

As we stand still on a rebounder, every cell in the body is opposing gravity. Your bathroom scale can be used as a "G" (gravity) meter. Place your bathroom scale on the rebounder and stand upon it. The scale registers one G force as long as you stand still. However, something fascinating happens when you start to move up and down. At the bottom of the bounce, you no longer weigh one G—you weigh *more* because the scale registers the combined forces of gravity *plus* deceleration when your body stops its downward thrust and acceleration when the expanded springs of the rebounder contract and force your body back up.

Acceleration + Deceleration + Gravity = Greater G Force! Even without allowing your feet to leave the rebounder mat, your G force increases to approximately 125%. It is vitally important to realize that *every* cell in your body is directly affected by that 25% increase in G force. Each cell is individually stressed by an increase of 25%.

If you ask a doctor, physical therapist, or coach for the formula to strengthen your cells, the answer would be, *"Controlled stress, below the rupture threshold, times repetition."* Bouncing on a rebounder stresses every cell over and over again approximately 100 times per minute. Remember, every cell in your body has the unique ability to automatically adjust to its environment. By stressing every cell over and over again, every cell will begin to adjust to a greater G force and thereby become stronger. If the word "stress" bothers you, think "exercise" instead. But this is one instance where "stress" is good for your body.

Other forms of exercise only oppose gravity, and thereby strengthen, *part* of your body. But if you oppose gravity with the added force of acceleration and deceleration created by rebounding, *you strengthen every cell in your body all at once.* This, in a nutshell and oversimplified, is the amazing theory of rebounding exercise. You can now begin to understand *why* rebounding has to be the most efficient, effective form of exercise yet devised by man.

There is three times more lymph fluid in the body than there is blood. What is "lymph?" Lymph is the clear fluid that oozes over a cut once it stops bleeding. Lymph is water, nutrients on the way to the cells, and waste by-products excreted from the cells for disposal. Lymph fluid is in constant motion around all cells. Our cells are able to function better with fresh lymph filled with a proper concentration of oxygen, glucose, certain electrolytes, amino acids, protein, essential fatty acids, carbohydrates and hormones. When these vital substances replace the waste products of the cells—the toxins, poisons, and trash that build up around inactive cells—we are healthier.

Because the lymph does not circulate with a pump system, as blood does, what moves it around? Lymph travels through our Auxiliary Circulating System, tubes whose cell walls are only one-cell thick. They reach nearly every part of the body. Where these tubes don't reach, there are minute passages where lymph can flow. The tiny lymph moves along a pressure hydraulic system. Pressure built up below the valve causes it to open. Pressure above the valve keeps it closed. An increase in pressure causes the lymph to flow upward.

The lymphatic system has the responsibility of pulling out waste, toxins, poisons, and extra-cellular trash from the body. Lymph fluid, filled with toxins, waste, excess protein and dead cellular particles, is sucked into the lymph tubes to be filtered by the spleen and the lymph nodes. The lymphatic system is our "vacuum cleaner," the garbage collector of the body.

Rebound exercise has been found the single most effective method of stimulating lymphatic circulation. Rebounding yields the greatest change in pressure for the least muscle effort. Why is that important? If our lymphatic system functions properly, we are healthy. If the lymph circulates improperly, we fall ill.

Every cell in the body is an "intelligent" entity in itself. Each cell has within its walls the complete blueprint of the entire body. Although every cell in the body owns its own copy of the blueprint, it only "reads" that part of the blueprint that has to do with its own function. A skin cell will always be a skin cell, a bone cell will always be a bone cell, and a liver cell will always be a liver cell.

Red blood cells, the most abundant of all the body's cells, are adept at transporting oxygen from the lungs to the tissues. Their function makes it necessary that they be able to move around the cardiovascular system without attachments. Red blood cells make up about 25% of all the body's cells.

Because every cell in the body has the ability to automatically adjust to its own environment, any change in the environment stimulates that cell or group of cells. Each cell is made strong by the amount and type of stimulation it receives. The stimulation put on a cell comes from three sources: (1) atmospheric or environmental pressure, (2) the gravitational pull of the earth, and (3) muscular activity. The greater the stimulation applied to the cell, the stronger it becomes as it adjusts to its environment.

Rebounder exercise is a method of stimulating every cell of the body simultaneously by increasing the G force applied to every cell. As we add the forces of acceleration and deceleration to gravity, every cell in the body begins to adjust automatically to its new environment.

MUSCLE STRENGTH & PHYSICAL FITNESS ARE NOT THE SAME—A study of the fitness, health and longevity of individuals over 100 years of age around the world, most of slight build best described as "wiry," revealed a very important common denominator. In every case, just getting through a normal day's work required great physical exertion. Using modern techniques, heart and lung function of these persons were monitored. Astoundingly enough, many of these people had "silent" cardiovascular diseases without exhibiting any of the usual symptoms, such as shortness of breath, and high blood pressure—but had not succumbed to a heart attack! The inescapable conclusion was that the seeming harshness of their daily lives stressed each cell constantly, resulting in an individual able to withstand a normally lethal heart attack!

Muscles are communities of cells with one main responsibility—to contract upon demand, thereby moving a bone or organ. Muscles get their strength from the combined total strength of their individual cells. In order to strengthen a muscle, the cells of that muscle must be strengthened individually.

Body-builders, for instance, concentrate on strengthening and building their muscles. *A muscle may be strong, but the individual may not be fit or healthy.* If the necessary oxygen and nutrients are not available when the cell needs them, or if there are too many toxins, wastes and poisons around the cells, it is impossible for the cell to function properly and the muscle will quickly become fatigued.

Many people mistake the terms "strength" and "physical fitness." Physical fitness is a measure of circulation efficiency. Increase the circulation efficiency of the body's fluids—the lymph and the blood—and the body is then physically fit and the muscles are able to continue to work longer without fatigue.

Rebounding not only increases the strength of each muscle by increasing the G force repeatedly, but also increases the fitness of the body by improving the lymphatic and blood circulation servicing the muscle. Unless your aim is bulging biceps, physical fitness is more important to most of us than mere muscle strength.

How in the world do you exercise an internal organ?—By rebounding to exercise the *cells* that make up the organ, of course. In the same way we strengthen muscle, we can build stronger, more efficient vital organs.

Various organs within the body are responsible for controlling the homeostatic condition of the environment for the individual cell. Many hundreds of control mechanisms are necessary to control arterial pressure, oxygen concentration, carbon dioxide concentration and the rates of individual chemical reactions in the individual cells. Each cell of each organ has to "do its own thing" without interfering with the function of cells within other organs. And each organ must work in harmony with the others.

All control systems of the body have certain characteristics in common. Most body organs function by reacting to opposition of their neutral position. For example, if the extra-cellular fluid becomes unbalanced, the system controlling a group of organs initiates the changes that cause an opposite reaction. This keeps the environment of the cells that comprise the organs near a certain concentration, maintaining the necessary balance.

The stimulation of the rapid vertical movement of the body on a rebounder causes all vital organs to work harder at controlling the body's environment. Because the rebounder has cured many physical problems, many people call it a "miracle machine." But the rebounder is not a miracle—the body is. The rebounder merely assists the body's organs to function more efficiently.

REBOUNDING IS AEROBICS, PLUS—*Aerobics* is the term used to define the function of cells that need oxygen to burn nutrients to create energy. All cells need oxygen and are therefore aerobic. Any activity, including sleeping, needs oxygen.

The body is unable to store oxygen, but we are able to replenish our supply simply by breathing. The problem is not *supplying* the body with oxygen—it is *delivering* oxygen to the cells where it is needed.

Exercise that elevates the heart-rate stimulates the pumping action of oxygen-carrying blood to all parts of the body. Aerobic exercise delivers greater amounts of oxygen to all cells more efficiently. In addition, increased demands on the body's arteries improves their elasticity. To transport blood effectively, our arteries must contract their inside diameters. But our arteries have a tendency to harden and become less elastic as we age, making the necessary contractions difficult. Aerobic exercise reverses this trend, causing arteries to become more elastic and easier to contract.

Rebounding / 15

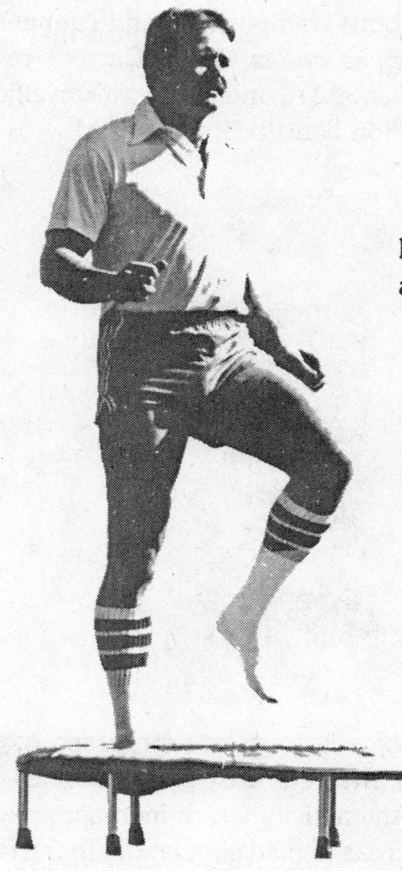

Randy Earl demonstrating the aerobic use of The Rebounder.

Who needs aerobic exercise? We all do—but not the level of exertion which often accompanies the better known aerobics such as walking, jogging, swimming, cycling and running. Many authorities caution that our bodies are not capable of coping with the shock and trauma caused by many of these activities.

However, the heart-rate drops after performing a good aerobic exercise for a few weeks. The heart muscle itself also increases in strength under controlled environmental stress, improving cardiac output. In other words, the heart can do more work with

16 / *Hidden Secrets of Super-Perfect Health*

each beat, or the same work with fewer beats. The average American has a resting pulse rate in the neighborhood of 75. As a case in point for aerobics, both trampolinists and runners are famous for having pulse rates as low as 45. (Al Carter's resting pulse rate has been recorded as 39.) An individual with an efficient heart saves about fifteen million heart-beats per year!

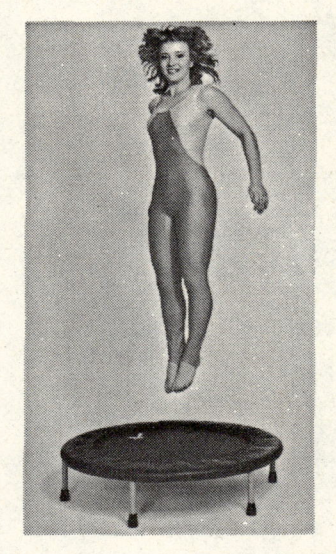

Wendie Carter
(Al's daughter)
Girls just wanna
have fun!

The premise behind aerobics is to create increased oxygen circulation to the cells. But the *real* answer is *aerobics plus increased fluid circulation*. Any activity which increases oxygen circulation will also cause increased fluid circulation. In the study of aerobics, the benefits appear to be caused by more efficient oxygen consumption, when, in fact, the benefits of aerobic activity are actually the result of a *combination* of better lymphatic circulation, better delivery of nutrients by the blood, more efficient oxygen utilization from the lungs and even better elimination and digestion because of more efficient body fluid circulation.

Studies conducted at the University of California show maximum cardiovascular efficiency can be achieved by rebounding aerobically for two four-minute periods daily.

Although it brings other benefits as well, rebounding for any longer than that will not improve heart efficiency noticeably. But the beauty of rebounding over running, the most popular aerobic exercise, is that rebounding doesn't foster "jogger's kidney," muscle strains, pulled ligaments or joint inflammation.

SURPRISE YOUR EYES—Who ever heard of exercising your eyes? In fact, most people are astounded to learn vision can be improved with exercise. We assume a person is born with "good" or "bad" eyes and nothing can be done about it. The idea of improving eyesight through exercise can be traced to the Egyptians, but we have become so convinced that we have no control over the condition of our eyes that we calmly accept the inconvenience.

You may be surprised to learn that the shape of the eyeball changes under stress, pressure, exercise, nutritional deficiencies, illness, shock or trauma. While examining over 30,000 eye patients per year, Dr. William W. Bates of the College of Physicians & Surgeons noticed some of his patients could see better on some occasions than others. He noted that farsightedness and near-sightedness came and went on some of his patients, *contrary to everything he had been taught.* This led him to the logical conclusion that the eyeball must be able to change shape and could be influenced by emotional stress, strain and exercise.

How do we exercise the eyes? Visual therapists have developed a number of eye exercises proven beneficial under specific circumstances and certainly any qualified ophthalmologist will be able to provide you with instruction. But where does rebounding fit into visual therapy? *The rebounder contributes more to the organization of visual perception than any other known device.* Our control of movement comes from the visual mechanism, because the eyes are the primary "steering" machinery for all movements. Improved vision comes about when the millions of cells in the eyes and the muscles controlling the eyes are individually stimulated to do a better job because of increased stress.

Try rebounding and "see" for yourself.

I Wanna Bounce

You have read the preceeding material with growing enthusiasm and now you're convinced that rebounding is the perfect exercise for you ... and you're right. Rebounding is so incredibly versatile it is the perfect exercise for everyone and everyone can benefit. It doesn't matter whether you're a great grandparent, an infant, or an athlete - or somewhere in between. Rebounding can be both gentle enough for a patient in a wheelchair and challenging enough for an athlete in training.

Rebounding is healthy exercise for the entire body, but a few cautions are in order. Injured cells, new cellular formations, aging cells, and cells weakened by disease or disuse have a very low threshold. Some elderly or extremely inactive people may experience pain or swelling in their weaker parts after rebounding. *This does not mean that rebound exercise is not good for them.* It merely means they should rebound with a gentler bounce, how gentle being determined by how weak their cells are. By *gradually* rebounding longer and harder, they will become stronger and increase their threshold to the point where they no longer have to worry about hurting something with the slightest amount of exercise.

Our bodies respond positively to challenge. The difference between our bodies and a mechanical device is that an automobile, for instance, deteriorates from wear and tear - but the body improves with use as long as the activity is not too violent.

When beginning any exercise program, be conservative. Do not over-exert yourself. Build endurance slowly. Rebound exercise is so easy that many beginners rebound too long the first time and feel it the next day. A consultation with your doctor is in order if you have any serious condition of ill health. However, rebounding is all it's said to be and the number of testimonials from enthusiastic rebounders is growing by leaps and bounds with glowing reports of ill health conquered.

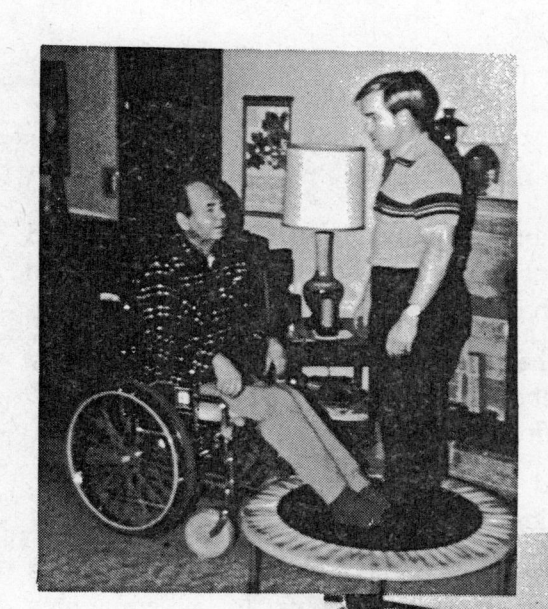

Al Carter (with Norman Nielson) demonstrating the early use of The Rebound with a wheelchair patient.

Al Carter (with Norman Nielson) demonstrating a more advanced program of rebounding for an incapacitated patient.

The Facts Of Life
Presented by Al Carter,
President of Rebound Dynamics, Inc.

FACT I.   Most rebound units are not built well enough to support a consistent exercise program longer than 30 days.

FACT II. NASA has confirmed to Al Carter personally that Rebound Exercise is as much as *68% more efficient* than jogging.

FACT III. Rebound Exercise is fun, easy, convenient, economical and safe for most people.

FACT IV. Al Carter's company, *Rebound Dynamics* has exclusive distribution rights to all copyrights owned by The National Institute of Reboundology & Health, which has published over 95% of all Rebound Exercise literature available.

FACT V.   Rebound Exercise helps improve body balance, coordination, rhythm, timing and dexterity, while building muscle strength.

FACT VI. Rebound Exercise is here to stay because it is *the most efficient and effective form of exercise yet devised by man.*

The Decline & Fall Of The Drugstore Rebounder

In 1979, Al Carter's first book, *Miracles of Rebound Exercise*, introduced rebounding to a wildly enthusiastic general public and sales skyrocketed. All those with the nose for a fast-buck jumped on the bandwagon and cheap, shoddy rebounders flooded the marketplace.

By 1980, there were over 100 manufacturers trying to cash-in on the rebound exercise industry. If the nylon mat looked like expensive permatron, customers couldn't tell the difference - until a half hour after they started bouncing. Some never did figure out why rebounding didn't seem to do much for them. The trouble is that nylon, like plastic and canvas, stretches. Most of these good people who thought they caught a bargain had simply never experienced rebounding on the right kind of equipment. They didn't know the difference between the sluggish thud of feet on their unit and the exhilarating free springing mat of a good unit.

Thin metal frames, cheap springs that stretched-out or snapped, and rubber leg tips that wore through in less than a month, damaging both floors or carpet, made it easy to reduce the price still more. Most people couldn't tell the difference in the store anyway.

Then the mass merchandisers entered the market in a big way, awarding a manufacturing contract to the lowest-bidder, of course. The mass merchandisers weren't knowledgeable enough on the health benefits of rebounding to understand the necessity of a quality unit. They just wanted a piece of the mini-trampoline market pie like everybody else. The main function of the mass merchandisers is to sell product to the masses - and, at $49.00 per unit, they succeeded.

The next entries came from foreign shores. Made with cheap materials and even cheaper labor, the foreign manufacturers stole the market with units retailing in drugstores and even some supermarkets at $19.95 and most of the U.S. manufacturers went out of business. The price war on rebounders that Al Carter predicted two years ago had finally run its course.

More than a million and a half rebounders were sold in 1983. These figures were up by more than 33% over 1982 when an astounding 72 million dollars were spent by consumers on rebounders! In 1984, department stores, discount stores, sporting goods stores and drugstores accounted for more than 78% of all sales of rebound units. These are the rebounders disgusted consumers pitched into the trash when the springs were sprung or the legs broke off or the mat split. The original and dedicated U.S. manufacturers responsible for starting the industry took only 13% of the sales volume. *Why?* Their actual construction costs were more than the cheap units' full retail price!

If you're one of the millions who got stuck with a piece of junk in the past and gave up on rebounding - or if you're new to this form of exercise - the best news of all is that Al Carter has personally supervised the design and construction of a rebounder which will meet or exceed the requirements of Certified Reboundologists all over the world! Called *The Rebound*, this unit retails for approximately $140 and is being manufactured in Taiwan in order to keep the price affordable.

Al tells us he has emphatically impressed on the factory that *quality* is essential. If manufactured in the U.S., the price would necessarily be approximately $250 retail for the same quality, but Al feels strongly it's vitally important to keep the cost of *The Rebound* within reach of all those who need it.

Al Carter has personally developed eleven specific exercises for the rebounder, one or more of them just right for you. Space considerations prevent our showing the pictures and instructions you will find in his book, but the titles of each will give you an idea of the wide range possible on *The Rebound*.

They are: (1) Health Exercise, (2) Aerobic Exercise, (3) Strength Exercise, (4) Twist, (5) Dance, (6) Slalom, (7) Goose Step, (8) Sitting, (9) Sitting with Assistance, (10) Wheel Chair Rebounding, and (11) The "V" Bounce.

Rebounding / 23

Mrs. Albert E. Carter (Bonnie) demonstrating the Health Exercise, a low bounce wherein the feet never leave the mat.

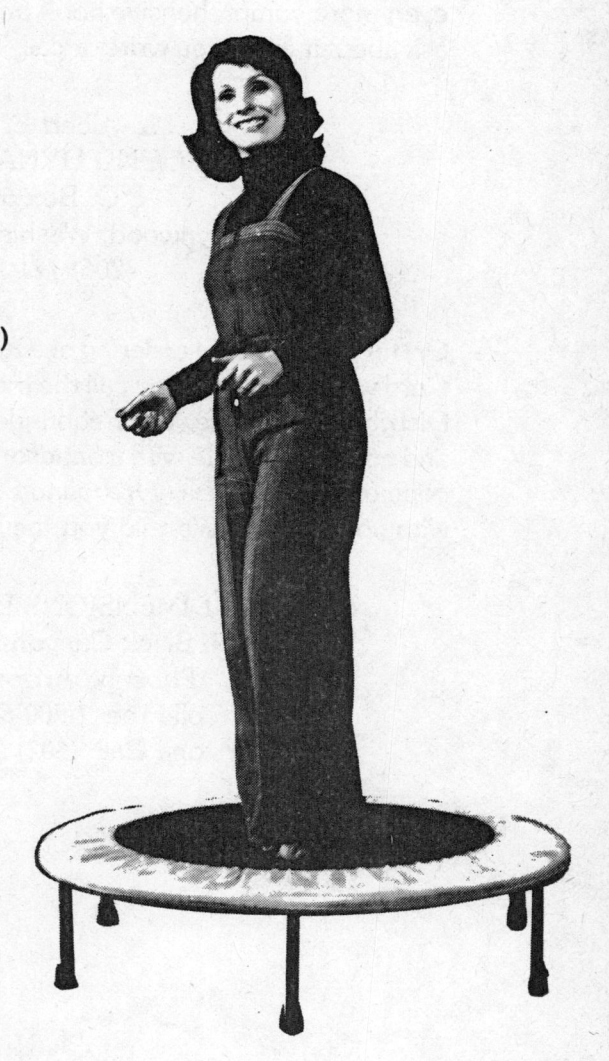

24 / Hidden Secrets of Super-Perfect Health

You will also find eye exercises, plus a method of improving memory, and an explanation of how trampolining is a positive aid to education in schools

You have nothing to lose but your aches and pains and excess weight. I strongly urge you to contact Al Carter for the name of your local Rebound distributor and to secure a copy of his book, *The Miracles of Rebound Exercise*. Incidentally, Al has another even more comprehensive book on rebounding in the works, so ask about it when you write or call. To contact Al, write or phone:

Mr. Albert E. Carter
REBOUND DYNAMICS, INC.
P.O. Box 5968F
Lynwood, Washington 98036
(206) 771-1462

Or, for fast and easy ordering of a Rebound unit (Visa and Master Card welcome), you may call the friendly folk at New Dimensions Distributors toll-free. The Rebounder folds in half for easy storage and comes complete with a handsome protective case. Special: A copy of *The Miracles of Rebound Exercise* will be included FREE with your order. (We told you they were friendly!)

NEW DIMENSIONS DISTRIBUTORS
2419 N. Black Canyon Highway, Suite 7
Phoenix, Arizona 85007
Call Toll-Free: 1-800-624-7114 Ext. 18
In Arizona Call: (602) 257-1183 Ext. 18

CHAPTER 2

Sweet, Crunchy, Juicy Carrots

This Familiar Vegetable Offers Great Health Benefits

ACROSS THE AGES—Carrots have been around a lot longer than you might think. The carrot (Daucus carota) is a native wild plant of the coastal regions of southern Europe and was widely cultivated by many ancient civilizations. Writing about the medicinal value of the plant, Pliny says: "The cultivated has the same virtues as the wild variety, although the latter is more powerful, especially when found growing in stony places."

Old herbals recommend the use of the seeds as well as the root. According to these writings, carrot seeds are very useful against gas, colic, hiccoughs, dysentery and chronic coughs. Carrot tea was considered a particularly valuable remedy for chronic kidney diseases and all afflictions of the bladder. Carrots have long been used in the treatment of dropsy (fluid retention). The name Carrot comes from the Celtic and means 'red of color'. Its botanical name, 'Daucus', is from the Greek *dais*, meaning 'to burn' and is representative of the carrot's stimulating qualities. One of the oldest surviving mentions of the carrot is in a Greek Cookbook written in 230 A.D.

The carrot was first introduced to England during the reign of Queen Elizabeth I by refugees fleeing from the persecutions of

Phillip II of Spain, as was its cousin, the parsnip. The carrot was immediately welcomed by the British peasantry and gentry alike. In the time of James I., aristocratic ladies of fashion used the feathery leaves as decoration in their elaborate hair-dresses. There is evidence that the carrot was grown in the U.S. in the Virginia colony as early as 1609.

Carrots Are Powerful Nutrition

THE 'EYE VITAMIN'—With its abundant Vitamin A (alpha and beta carotene), often called 'the eye vitamin', the carrot is one of the very best aids for strengthening poor vision. The story of Elizabeth K., a young mother of two, very clearly illustrates what the lowly carrot can do in the case of night-blindness arising as a consequence of a deficiency of Vitamin A.

This young woman arranged her life so that she would never have to drive at night. Her night-blindness was very severe and she feared being behind the wheel from dusk on, recognizing her inability to see clearly under these conditions. But, as luck would have it, her husband was off on a business trip when one of the children went into convulsions. The young mother was terrified and bundled both little ones into the car and started off for the hospital at 15 miles per hour. She arrived without incident and the child was successfully treated. But Elizabeth realized that she must do something about her night-blindness because, in an emergency, she might be forced to drive at night and the next time might not be so fortunate.

The following day, Elizabeth bought a juicer and began juicing and drinking a full quart of fresh carrot juice every day. Her husband joked that she was 'turning yellow', but she persisted and even served each member of the family a glass of carrot juice at breakfast. After only a few weeks, Elizabeth found her night-blindness was clearing. She continued on her self-imposed regimen and now drives at night with complete confidence.

General Health Benefits

VITAMINS & MINERALS—Carrots provide an ample supply of beta-carotene and Vitamins A, B, C, D, E, G, and K. They are appreciated for their healthy vitamin and mineral content and are very easy on the digestive tract.

Carrots are particularly rich in potassium and offer a goodly quantity of calcium, magnesium, iron, phosphorous, and sulphur. These vital alkaline elements are perfectly balanced in carrots and aid the body in many important functions.

THE DINNER TABLE MEDICINAL—Because carrots are easily assimilated, a puree of raw carrots is often recommended by naturally-oriented pediatricians to correct gastric disturbances in very young children and to improve digestion in general. Carrots are mildly diuretic, strengthen the immune system, reinforce eyesight and aid in correcting all gastro-intestinal disorders in adults and children alike. Carrots act to improve resistance to infections of all types, especially of the eyes, throat and tonsils, as well as the sinuses and the entire respiratory system.

The nutrients present in carrots stimulate the vital endocrine glands, protect the nervous system, and are unequalled for increasing vim, vigor, and vitality. The glands, particularly the adrenals and the hormone-secreting glands of the reproductive system, require the food elements found in carrots. Because certain forms of sterility have been traced to the over-use of over-processed foods in which vital nutrients and enzymes were destroyed, carrots have been known to overcome sterility.

Intestinal and liver complaints are often caused by a deficiency of certain elements known to be supplied by carrots. These elements act to dissolve and free unhealthy toxins clogging the system, releasing them for excretion.

For gastrointestinal catarrh, naturalists recommend you finely grate one pound of carrots, saute lightly, and dilute with half a cup of good broth. Take nothing else for the entire day. This cleansing treatment is a great help in normalizing digestion and aids the kidneys.

Carrots are particularly good as a supportive treatment for diabetics and including carrots regularly in the diet may help ease the pain of gout, rheumatism and arthritis. Premature hair loss, if caused by a vitamin deficiency, may yield to strong, regular use of grated or juiced carrots as well.

CANCER—With their important content of beta-carotene (a precursor of Vitamin A), new research indicates that carrots may have preventive and even curative powers in the case of cancer, particulary of the lungs. The cancer-preventive properties of beta-carotene are stronger than those of Vitamin A itself. The powerful difference between the two is that beta-carotene carries a mysterious type of live electrical charge, while Vitamin A does not. Another important difference is that beta-carotene has little harmful effect on the liver.

As both a preventive and an active cancer treatment, beta-carotene has been shown to effectively destroy the cancer cell's protective layer of mucus, opening it to the body's natural defense mechanisms. Proponents of beta-carotene predict reduction in the rate of certain forms of cancer for those who regularly include carrots in their diet (up to 80 percent of cancer in the lungs and bronchia, and up to 55 percent in cancer of the colon). Carrots are the single most important source of beta-carotene in nature. This common garden vegetable is considered the first line of defense as a cancer preventive of the highest order.

It is important to note that beta-carotene is fat-soluble and can only be absorbed and assimilated by the body in the presence of a fatty emulsion. The essential fatty acids the body requires are present in butter and cream, but a daily regimen which includes linseed oil and cottage cheese may be a healthier way to ingest these fats. (See *Linseed Oil,* Chapter 6.)

Raw carrot juice is considered a natural solvent for all ulcers and cancerous conditions. Many naturopathic doctors suggest that smokers and those with a family history of cancer may benefit by adding a cup of raw carrots or freshly squeezed carrot juice to their daily diet. Some authorities believe the preventive powers of this dietary supplement may also apply to internal ulcers.

SKIN DISCOLORATION—It is not the beta-carotene or the orange coloring of carrots which tints the skin. You don't turn 'green' after eating green vegetables or 'red' after eating beets or 'orange' after eating carrots (or squash or apricots).

Like the young mother who conquered night-blindness with vast quantities of carrot juice, an intensive treatment with carrots may tend to impart a yellowish-orange tint to the skin. If this happens to you, rejoice! The condition is temporary and shows that so many toxins are being leached out of the body that the overflow is being released through the pores of the skin.

The elements in carrots assist in detoxifying and cleansing the liver, one of the body's most important organs. If the normal eliminative passageways (intestines and urinary tract) are insufficient to carry it all away, the remainder is released through the skin. As a matter of fact, the skin itself is the largest eliminative organ of the body.

How To Enjoy Carrots

COOKED—Carrots may be lightly cooked, but the medicinal vitamins and mineral elements are much greater in the fresh state. If you just can't enjoy carrots without cooking, remember that steaming retains a great deal more of the important vitamin and mineral content than does old-fashioned boiling.

Slivered carrots are a delightful addition to any stir-fry dish. When prepared in this traditional oriental manner and allowed to remain crunchy, very little of carrot's healthy benefits are lost.

RAW—Well-masticated (chewed) raw carrots and grated raw carrots are equally effective, so take your choice. But please grate only what you plan on eating immediately. Grated carrots must be eaten the same day.

JUICED—Scrub, but don't peel, a quantity of raw carrots and run them through your juicer. The properties of carrot juice are strongest when taken immediately, so please don't hold the juice refrigerated, but enjoy it when prepared.

CARROT CEREAL—For each serving, soak 1/2 cup of Oat Flakes in cold milk overnight. The following morning, add a finely grated carrot. Warm slightly, sweeten with honey, and be fortified with carrot-power for the day.

CARROT JAM—Scrub, but don't peel, a quantity of carrots under cold-running water. Grate finely, add enough water to barely cover, and simmer over low heat until you have a fine pulp. For each 2 cups of pulp, add the juice and grated rind of two lemons, 1/2 stick of butter, and 9 ounces of sugar. Simmer the mixture until the consistency of jam, about 40 minutes. Bottle in clear glass and store refrigerated.

No matter how you choose to include the lowly carrot in your diet, be sure to do it. Carrots offer unparalleled health and nutritive benefits of the highest order. I'm betting that once you try a glass of freshly prepared carrot juice, you'll find it so tasty and refreshing that you won't even realize that you're sipping nature's finest 'preventive medicine.'

EDITOR'S NOTE: This chapter comprises an excerpt in its entirety from *Miracle Healing Power Through Nature's Pharmacy* (Fischer Publishing Company, Canfield, Ohio 44406). Even though this material duplicates material published in the foregoing book, the decision to include this chapter in this book was taken by the author because of the importance of the material.

CHAPTER 3

Vitamin P — The Naturalist's Vitamin

Together Forever: Vitamin P (The Bioflavonoids) & Vitamin C

IN THE BEGINNING—It was Scottish naval surgeon James Lind who proved that scurvy, the leading cause of disease and death afflicting seamen on long sea voyages, could be prevented simply by providing fresh fruit to the sailors. In 1753 when Dr. Lind made this momentous discovery, Vitamin C was unnamed and unknown. It wasn't until the late 1920s that Dr. Albert Szent-Gyorgyi, the renowned Hungarian physician and scientist, succeeded in isolating Vitamin C (for citrus) from oranges. Most authorities were content to believe that Vitamin C was the sole active element in citrus fruits. But, after a period of nine years in clinical use, it was determined that ascorbic acid (Vitamin C) alone just wasn't very effective against certain conditions of ill health.

In the meantine, Dr. Szent-Gyorgyi had continued work in his laboratory. The good doctor won the Nobel prize in 1936 when he discovered a group of additional elements in fresh lemons and green peppers. When these additional elements were given to patients along *with* Vitamin C, the patients responded more favorably than when given Vitamin C alone.

Vitamin P

THE BIOFLAVONOIDS—It is because these elements exercise a strengthening effect on the permeability of the capillaries, the tiniest blood vessels, that they are named Vitamin P. Scientifically speaking, Vitamin P consists of a group of natural *flavone glycosides*, or bioflavonoids. So far, researchers have separated out and identified rutin, hesperidin, and citrin as bioflavonoids, but there may be more.

Although many fresh fruits and certain vegetables are good sources of the bioflavonoids, you won't get them in jams, juices, or casseroles. Bioflavonoids are largely destroyed by cooking and it is the white pulpy part (in vegetables and fruits) and the thin skin separating the sections in citrus that provides the Vitamin P.

However, the most important thing you must understand is this: In nature, Vitamin C and Vitamin P are found together. They work synergistically within the body. In other words, each activates the other and together they are more potent and powerful than either is alone.

THE FUNCTIONS OF VITAMIN P—Bioflavonoids are essential for the efficient absorption and assimilation of Vitamin C. They also work with Vitamin C to keep collagen healthy. Collagen represents about 30 percent of the total protein content of the body. It is an important element of cellular connective tissue, promotes youthful elasticity of the skin, and is a vital part of ligaments, cartilage, and bone.

The bioflavonoids increase the strength of the capillaries and regulate their permeability. These actions help prevent hemorrhages and ruptures of the capillaries and cellular connective tissues. Vitamin P also assists the immune system in fighting infection and bacterial invasion by foreign substances.

Like Vitamin C, the bioflavonoids are water-soluble and readily absorbed from the gastrointestinal tract into the bloodstream. They have no known upper limits of ingestion, exhibit no toxicity, and any excess is excreted through urination and perspiration.

World – Wide Research

WHAT'S GOING ON—The brotherhood of scientists around the world has been conducting extensive research on the properties of Vitamin P for close to three decades. Results of clinical tests on the preventive and therapeutic uses of the bioflavonoids have been published in respected medical journals world-wide.

The U.S.S.R. — A symposium of Soviet scientists investigated bioflavonoids and, in a report entitled *Vitamin P—Its Properties & Its Uses,* revealed the successful treatment of many diseases. The Russian report particulary stressed the capillary strengthening effects of bioflavonoids.

Approximately 32 percent of laboratory mice injected with a virulent strain of influenza and treated with Vitamin P survived, while almost 90 percent of the mice in the untreated control group died of the flu virus.

Good results were obtained when treating patients suffering from high blood pressure (hypertension) with bioflavonoids. The Russian researchers noted that blood pressure rose again when the treatment was discontinued.

SWITZERLAND—Targeting the decongestive action of Vitamin P, the Medical Polyclinic of the University of Geneva states they have treated thousands of patients suffering from hemorrhoids with Vitamin P4 (*bioflavonoid trioxyethylrutin*). Pain, itching, and burning were relieved and often the hemorrhoids completely disappeared.

The Dermatological Clinic of the University of Lausanne calls Vitamin P4 the first important advance in the treatment of varicose veins and other venous diseases in years. Of the 1400 patients suffering with hemorrhoids, varicose veins, inflammation of the capillaries, and chronic venous insufficiency, 1100 showed fair to good results after ingestion of Vitamin P4.

AUSTRALIA—Australian M.D.s W.C. Martin and M.S. Biskind reported a 90 percent success rate treating colds, flu, and tonsillitis with bioflavonoids. Most patients made a dramatic full recovery within eight hours after ingesting Vitamin P. The physicians determined that oral ingestion of the bioflavonoids was effective no matter how long the condition had persisted prior to treatment.

THE U.S.—The American Journal of Gastroenterology reported on 36 patients suffering with bleeding duodenal ulcers who were treated with bioflavonoids. A mixture of orange juice, milk, and gelatin was given along with Vitamin P every two hours until the bleeding stopped. All bleeding was arrested within four days and all patients responded favorably. By the end of the 22 day course of therapy, duodenal contours had returned to normal and the mucous membranes had fully regenerated.

Dr. James R. West, of the Morrell Memorial Hospital in Lakeland, Florida, treated a woman in her mid-fifties with bioflavonoids for her rheumatoid arthritis. The unfortunate woman was afflicted in both hands, wrists, elbows, knees, ankles, and her right shoulder. After two weeks, the pain had all but been eliminated and her blood pressure dropped to a healthy 136. After five weeks, her joints were moving more freely and she had a great deal more stamina.

MORE RESULTS—Vitamin P has been shown useful in the treatment of bleeding gums, eczema, and a tendency to hemorrhage. Asthmatics have been helped with bioflavonoids and Vitamin P appears to exert a protective effect against the harm that x-rays can cause as well. *Labyrinthitis,* a condition of the inner ear canal which affects balance and causes extreme dizziness, has been successfully treated with Vitamin P.

When Vitamin C and P are administered together, the combination may assist in preventing miscarriage. Both rheumatism and rheumatic fever succumb and a blood vessel disorder of the eye which often afflicts diabetics may be helped as well. Because bioflavonoids have been useful in reducing high blood pressure, they may be of moderate assistance in cases of muscular dystrophy.

Both weekend warriors and professional athletes should know that bioflavonoids are beneficial in treating capillary injuries and act to minimize the unavoidable bruising that occurs in some sports.

NOTE: Because Mother Nature provides Vitamin C and P in precisely the right combination in fresh foods (and Mother knows best), any bioflavonoid preparation will be synergistically potentiated and results heightened with the addition of ascorbic acid (Vitamin C).

Food Sources Of Vitamin P

COMMON FOODS—Excellent sources of the important bioflavonoids (with Vitamin C) include all the citrus fruits, grapes, plums, currants, apricots, cherries, blackberries, green peppers, and buckwheat. Just remember that there is ten times the concentration of Vitamin P in the edible part of the fruit than there is in juice.

ROSE HIPS—Knowledgeable nutritionists around the world recognize that rose hips contain thirty times more Vitamin C than oranges and are an extremely rich source of Vitamin P as well. Many healthful herbal tea blends contain rose hips as a prime ingredient. Rose hips may also be purchased powdered or tableted and some health food stores stock the whole 'vitamin rose' itself.

Vitamin P As A Preventive

To strengthen the entire venous system, especially the fragile capillaries, nothing beats the bioflavonoids. Because many viral and bacterial infections, along with certain degenerative conditions (arthritis, cardiovascular disorders) are associated with weakened capillaries, the strengthening effects of Vitamin P become obviously important. Bruises and wounds heal faster with adequate stores of Vitamin P and it assists the immune system as well.

Along with Vitamin C, Vitamin P is an invaluable agent in the fight to prevent and/or correct many conditions of ill health. And it's just so easy (and pleasant) to eat some fresh fruit every day. Mind your P's and C's and feel better—naturally!

CHAPTER 4

Taking A Look At White Sugar

Is It Really A Major Health Hazard?

IN THE BEGINNING—As far back as 3000 B.C., India was making sugar, then called *guara*. The sweet stuff was considered so precious that the *Atharvaveda*, a sacred book of the Hindus (800 B.C.), describes a royal crown fashioned of sugar cane. In the 4th century B.C., a general under the command of Alexander the Great described a wondrous reed (sugar cane) which "produces honey without the aid of bees."

In Sanskrit, the ancient language of India, sugar is *sakara* (sand). Sugar making progressed from India to Arabia (*sukkar*), thence to Greece (*sakharon*), on to Italy (*zucchero*), across southern Europe into France (*sucre*), until it finally made its way to English dinner tables as *sugar*. By 1544, two sugar refineries were established in London.

Christopher Columbus is credited with bringing sugar cane to the New World on his second voyage in 1493. Because of the kind climate, sugar plantations immediately flourished in Santo Domingo and other islands of the West Indies. By 1689, sugar refining had begun in New York, one of the earliest of the American colonies. Sugar planting was attempted in Louisiana in 1737, but the plantations were not really successful until 1791, more than fifty years later.

It is interesting to note that sugar was originally considered a powerful medicinal. Ancient physicians dispensed it in tiny measures as a tranquilizer and sedative. It was not until the 17th century that sugar was used as a food or food sweetener. This scarce luxury was very expensive and few households could afford the use of it at all. As an indication of the high value placed on the sweet commodity in 1736, common table sugar was listed among the precious gems and art objects fashioned of costly metals given as wedding gifts to Maria Theresa, the future queen of Hungary.

TODAY—Table sugar can be purchased for around fifty cents per pound and is a staple in almost every home in America. Each and every person in the U.S. consumes, on average, close to 150 pounds of the sweet white crystals every year. In fact, 70 percent of that 150 pounds (about 105 pounds) is consumed by a heedless public in manufactured foods.

A vast array of commercially processed foods contain some form of sugar. It hides in places where you might not suspect its presence, including many no-salt spice blends, pastas, canned vegetables, vegetable juices, and even gravy mixes. It's hard to understand just *why*. I don't know anyone who deliberately dresses crisp, delicious garden vegetables with sugar or dumps sugar into meat juices while making gravy or sprinkles a teaspoon of sugar on pizza.

Dr. D.M. Hegsted, Professor of Nutrition, Harvard School of Public Health, was quoted in 1977 as saying, "The diet we eat today was not planned or developed for any particular purpose. It is a happenstance related to our affluence, the productivity of our farmers, and the activities of our food industry. The risks associated with eating this diet are demonstrably large."

Considering the proliferation of processed food products that have been developed in the last decade, we can only assume that the problem has been compounded over time. There are more manufactured foods in any supermarket today that there are foods in the form nature intended - and far too many of them contain needless sugar.

All Sugars Are Not The Same

GLUCOSE—When we eat food (carbohydrates), it is true that the body sorts out all the elements and eventually breaks down the constituents into simple sugars (glucose and fructose). Glucose is the major sugar present in blood and body tissue. This is an essential sugar in that all cells, especially brain cells, depend on glucose. But there is no RDA (Recommended Daily Allowance) for any kind of sugar, including glucose. We are not required to eat a measure of glucose every day. The specialized enzymes of the digestive tract are equipped to convert carbohydrates into the basic glucose the body needs.

Digestion begins the moment we put food into our mouths. Saliva contains special enzymes which begin processing carbohydrates into simple sugars as we chew. The digestive and assimilation process continues in the stomach and proceeds in the small intestine as pancreatic juices are introduced.

Glucose is the energy source the body needs. Glucose is released slowly into the bloodstream during the metabolic process, along with other needed nutrients.

SUCROSE—When we discuss sugar in this chapter, we are talking of sucrose, the white table sugar processed from sugar cane or sugar beets. One of the most common misconceptions today, fostered by some excellent advertising, is that sugar provides quick energy and is a good food. The catch is that sugar is not absorbed and metabolized in the body in the same efficient way as complex carbohydrates are.

When we eat sugar, it is rapidly absorbed and passed onto the liver where it is converted into triglycerides. The triglycerides are released into the blood stream and end up being stored as fat deposits in the veins and tissues. Do we have to remind you that high cholesterol and triglyceride levels are implicated in the development of cancer, heart disease, and many other life-threatening conditions?

An intake of sugar also triggers the release of insulin by the pancreas. The insulin metabolizes the sugar rapidly in order to maintain normal blood-sugar levels. But the sugar is digested and assimilated so quickly that a lot of excess insulin (with a much longer half-life than sugar) continues racing around the bloodstream and is left with nothing to process. This is the big reason why sugar picks you up fast, but lets you down even faster. Sugar is not a source of sustained energy at all.

It is obvious that the ingestion of large amounts of sugar over a long period of time places a tremendous stress on the pancreas. Diabetes results when the pancreas is exhausted and loses its ability to synthesize insulin. Diabetes (and related side effects) rank third (after heart disease and cancer) as a cause of death in America.

Classic Symptoms Of Sugar Toxicity

ADDICTION—Mrs. Bethine G., a personal friend of mine who holds a responsible position with a major airline, had a severe addiction to sugar. This 50-years (plus) career woman kept a bag of jelly beans (artificially flavored) in her desk and munched constantly. During a typical day, she drank black coffee from the time she got up until she went to bed. In the morning when she arrived at work, she ate a doughnut or two (containing sugar). Lunch was very often a soft drink (containing sugar), a sandwich of cold cuts (containing sugar) on white bread (refined carbohydrates). For dessert, Bethine generally selected a cream pie (both sugar and refined carbohydrates). Unless she went out to dinner, the evening 'meal' was usually an extended series of sweet nibbling on whatever came to hand at the end of a long day.

Over an extended period of time, Bethine became aware that she did not feel at all well. Her arms, feet, and legs were always numb and she complained of a constant 'tingling' feeling. She had such severe stomach cramps that she occasionally cried aloud and doubled over in pain. She was very often nauseous. She was always tired and was becoming apathetic. She had violent mood swings, laughing and joking one minute, crying the next, and then switching with lightening speed to a cool sarcastic mood. It was when she began suffering blurred vision and seeing double that she finally went to the doctor with her list of complaints.

After an extensive series of tests (blood, urinalysis, six-hour glucose tolerance test, and more), the doctor was satisfied that he had checked her out thoroughly. The diagnosis: Nothing physical was wrong. He hinted at stress and nervous exhaustion, but Bethine rejected the idea that her mind was making her body betray her somehow. She was convinced her symptoms were real and knew, in a vague sort of way, that they were related. She was at her wits end when she opened a popular publication and saw the word SUGAR printed across the page in bold, black headlines. As she read the accompanying article, Bethine realized that she was suffering the classic symptoms of sugar addiction.

Armed with this new knowledge, she went ruthlessly through her kitchen cupboards and read every label. She was amazed at the number of common processed foods that contained sugar on the ingredient panel. She passed up the doughnuts at work, tossed out a half eaten bag of her favorite jelly beans, and begun to select foods with high nutrient value.

Once Bethine eliminated sugar from her diet, was she miraculously cured? Yes and no. For a full seven days and more, she suffered withdrawal symptoms that might have deterred one less determined. Even though she ate fruit (containing healthy glucose) with a voracious appetite, she craved processed sweets (sucrose) with a passion. She had 'the shakes.' Her body temperature varied between cold and hot. Worst of all, she itched ferociously, She felt as if she had tiny bugs crawling all over her, but she persevered.

All this happened about ten months ago. Today, Bethine says she's healthier than she's ever been. She feels on top of the world, has more energy than her son or daughter, has lost over twenty pounds, and sparkles with vitality. It's now a pleasure to converse with this dynamic lady. As a friend, I am delighted to see this very real transformation.

If you still entertain a doubt that sugar is a toxic poison that can ruin your health, or that the overconsumption of sugar and refined carbohydrates builds a dependency that escalates into a true addiction, ask Bethine. She doesn't even miss it.

HYPOGLYCEMIA—She had all the symptoms. Miss Shelley H. was seventeen years old and no one knew what to do with her. Was it just a phase she was going through, or was she the victim of some deep undiscovered psychological trauma? This very attractive young lady couldn't sleep. She was constantly depressed, had anxiety attacks, was irritable in the extreme, and cried helplessly much of the time. Shelly suffered violent headaches and her back ached constantly. She complained that all her muscles ached. Her heart beat so fast sometimes that it frightened her. She didn't want to eat, couldn't sleep, her hands trembled, and she was so dizzy she sometimes bumped into furniture.

After a six-hour glucose tolerance test, the doctor confirmed that Shelley was suffering from *hypoglycemia*, or low blood sugar. Hypoglycemia is caused by an overdose of insulin, medically termed *hyperinsulinism*, or insulin shock. This condition arises because the pancreas secretes excessive insulin in response to an overconsumption of sugar.

Hypoglycemia is the opposite of diabetes. In hypoglycemia, the pancreas produces too much insulin and lowers the blood sugar levels rapidly. In diabetes, the pancreas does not produce sufficient insulin, or has become so exhausted trying to deal with excessive sugar that it can no longer secrete the insulin required to maintain normal blood sugar levels at all.

Shelley's doctor put her on a very carefully regulated diet. She responded within a few days to the elimination of sugar and refined carbohydrates and has learned to enjoy wholesome nutritious foods. For about four months, Shelly ate at least six small meals every day. She learned to manage her complex carbohydrate intake so skillfully that she no longer has to worry about counting grams and keeping a good balance.

This young woman is once again the very picture of health. She is now married, is raising three lovely daughters, and works part-time because she enjoys it. Her energy levels are high; her disposition is sunny. Shelly likes 'fussing' in the kitchen and prepares fresh foods almost exclusively. The entire family is thriving and Shelley is determined that no one within the sound of her voice will ever have to undergo the miseries of hypoglycemia. She preaches the dangers of sugar and refined carbohydrates far and wide. Those who see her immense vitality and glowing health listen and learn. She's an excellent 'advertisement' for natural eating.

Saccharine Disease

MORE — Saccharine disease is not related to the consumption of the artificial sweetener known as *saccharine*. Eating a diet high in refined carbohydrates results in what nutritionists call *saccharine disease*. Many breakfast cereals, cookies, cakes, pies, doughnuts (all made with refined white flour and overloaded with white sugar), soft drinks, and a lot of other commercially processed foods are examples of refined carbohydrates. Refined carbohydrate foods offer empty calories, very little fiber, and generally have an extremely low nutritive value.

SYMPTOMS OF SACCHARINE DISEASE - The overconsumption of refined carbohydrate foods results in physical problems such as chronic headaches, dental decay, constipation, obesity, ulcers, various skin conditions (hives, rashes, itching, swelling), hemorrhoids, varicose veins, Escherichia coli infections (diverticulitis, appendicitis, cholecystitis, pyelitis, renal calculus), hypoglycemia (a blood-sugar imbalance), metabolic disorders, diabetes, colitis, coronary heart disease, atherosclerosis, and even cancer. Over-consumption of refined carbohydrate foods involves the central nervous system as well, resulting in escalating tension, anxiety, depression, mood-swings (thought disorders, changes in behavior) and even hallucinations.

The excessive (and obsessive) eating of refined carbohydrates can be a very real addiction, as real as any addiction to alcohol or narcotics. As in any addiction, supplying the body with its daily 'fix' of sugar is done at the expense of foods with a high nutritive value. The end result is a form of malnutrition.

If you doubt that sugar is addictive, you should know that true sugar addicts who go 'cold-turkey' and eliminate sugar from their diet abruptly suffer the same type of withdrawal symptoms as do drug addicts. The experts say that eliminating sugar from the diet is best done slowly over a period of time.

DIABETES - Sir Frederick Banting, the man who discovered insulin, necessarily studied diabetes very carefully. His work provides a perfect and very well documented example of eating processed sugar and refined carbohydrates compared to the ingestion of complex carbohydrates.

While doing his research, Banting traveled to Panama, one of the world's sources of sugar, to observe the cane cutters in action. Typically, these laborers chewed on raw sugar cane all day long, but they had a very low incidence of diabetes as a group.

On the other hand, the plantation masters consumed as much pure processed white suger as the workers did cane. But, as a group, the employers who consumed pure sugar and ate a diet high in other refined carbohydrates as well, suffered a very high rate of diabetes indeed.

Banting observed that the cane cutters supplied their bodies with sugar slowly. While they were sucking and chewing the cane, they ingested some healthy fiber and vitamins and minerals along with the sugar in the cane. In contrast, the plantation masters who ate refined carbohydrates and processed white sugar were ingesting empty calories and foods with very little nutritive value.

NutraSweet®

Because so many consumers are switching to artificially sweetened products, we are including an update here on what's new in the NutraSweet controversy. NutraSweet is a 'hot item' right now. It seems that just about every manufacturer looking for an artificial sweetener has switched to NutraSweet. Aspartame, or NutraSweet, is an extremely popular low-calorie sweetener that the developer (Searle & Co.) claims is as natural as bananas with milk.

One of the major ingredients of NutraSweet is *phenylalanine,* an amino acid. Dr. Richard J. Wurtman of the Massachusetts Institute of Technology suggests that consuming large amounts of phenylalanine-laced NutraSweet can raise the levels of the chemical phenylalanine in the brain, thus interfering with the body's production of important neurotransmitters that protect against seizures.

RELATED HEALTH PROBLEMS — Dr Wurtman, publishing in the well respected British journal *Lancet,* cites three cases of individuals suffering their first epileptic seizures after drinking large quantities of beverages sweetened with NutraSweet.

A legal secretary who drank diet soda and lemonade containing NutraSweet all day long reported mood changes, headaches, nausea and hallucinations. She finally experienced a grand mal seizure that put her in the hospital.

A computer programmer who drank four to five glasses of a powdered drink sweetened with NutraSweet every day suffered abnormal breathing, night twitching, severe headaches, and a debilitating seizure.

A young college professor who drank a quart or more of NutraSweet sweetened iced tea had a seizure while sleeping.

These are not isolated occurrences either. Across the country, more and more individuals are discovering that they experience disturbing symptoms ranging from mild to severe while taking

NutraSweet or NutraSweet sweetened commercial products.

G.D. Searle & Co. has succeeded in popularizing NutraSweet through a systematic multi-million dollar advertising campaign. It is now widely used in diet drinks, chewing gum, puddings, and other products. (In the presence of excessive heat, such as in warehouse storage, NutraSweet can transform itself into methyl alcohol, a poisonous solvent which can cause loss of sight.) The big attraction of NutraSweet appears to be because it is perceived to be an "easy way" to lose weight while still enjoying the sweet taste that many dieters crave.

Even though the symptoms of NutraSweet poisoning usually disappear within a few weeks of eliminating the artificial sweetener from the diet, why risk your good health?

Sugar vs Other Natural Sweeteners

SUGAR AS A NUTRIENT—The nutritive value of white sugar is a big fat zero. It is a major carbohydrate source, but offers no amino acids (protein), vitamins or minerals. In order for the body to process and assimilate sugar, it must be supplied with B vitamins obtained from other foods (or in a pill). Sugar provides empty calories only. It is totally devoid of the essential components of a food.

MOLASSES AS A NUTRIENT—Plain ordinary molasses is a good vitamin and mineral source. It offers a measurable amount of vitamins (including Vitamin E) and minerals and is especially rich in iron, calcium, copper, magnesium, phosphorus, pantothenic acid, and inositol.

This sticky old-time sweetener can range in color from a very light to a very dark brown. Blackstrap molasses, with its strong metallic taste, is the thick residue remaining after every molecule of sugar has been extracted.

A Special Word About Honey

HONEY AS A NUTRIENT—Honey is a true energy food and is primarily a carbohydrate source in very easily digested form. This sweet from the beehive can be very rich in vitamins, minerals, and important nutrients in the raw state. However, filtered and refined honey has had all the minute bee pollen particles removed and has therefore lost a lot of its food value. For a healthy sweet, choose the cloudy unfiltered variety rather than the clear honey so common in supermarkets everywhere. Better yet, if you know a beekeeper, purchase your honey supply direct, when the beekeeper is extracting.

Honey is a lot sweeter than table sugar and less is needed to achieve the same degree of sweetness. Cooking with honey is especially rewarding. Using honey instead of sugar when baking, for instance, helps keep the end product moist and also acts as a natural preservative.

HONEY AS A HEALER—Honey has been prized as both a medicine and a sweetener since time began. Over 2000 years ago, Egyptian physicians called honey the "universal healer." In ancient China, honey was used to treat the victims of smallpox. The sticky stuff was smoothed over the entire body of the infected person. From all reports, this highly contagious and disfiguring disease was stopped in its tracks and no pitting or scarring ensued.

Science is now beginning to find out why this natural sweet is such good preventive medicine and how it benefits the body. The U.S Bureau of Entomology has discovered that honey kills harmful bacteria. When typhoid germs and dysentery germs are placed in a lab dish with a bit of raw honey, the dreaded typhoid is destroyed in 48 hours and the dysentery bacteria is destroyed in less than 10 hours. Honey is a powerful germ killer.

In Britain, researchers have verified what the healers of old knew very well. Doctors working at England's Norfold & Norwich

Hospital use raw honey to treat infected wounds with notable success. In days of old, honey was used to dress battle wounds.

A local farm wife of my acquaintance healed her husband of a deep ulcer on his right leg with honey. This man, George G., is a diabetic and developed a sore on his right leg. As is common in diabetics, the sore refused to heal. His doctors used all the resources at their command, but the sore ulcerated and became deeper and deeper until the very bone was affected. Nasty-smelling pus continually discharged from this ulcer. Amputation was discussed, but George resisted.

His wife, Maggie, finally remembered her grandmother using honey to speed the healing of open wounds. Figuring they had nothing to lose, Maggie began dressing George's ugly supperating ulcer with honey. Within a week, the wound seemed cleaner and stopped discharging pus. A month later, much to the astonishment of George's physician, the ulcer was healing normally. Although a deep depression in the flesh of George's right leg remains to show where the ulcer used to be, his leg is now strong and healthy.

Old-Time Honey Remedies

HONEY/LEMON COUGH SYRUP—Mix together equal parts of raw honey and freshly-squeezed lemon juice. Take one tablespoon as needed for a simple cough. Soothes and coats the throat.

GRANDMOTHER'S COUGH SYRUP—Add 1 tablespoon each glycerine (may be purchased at any drug store) and lemon (or lime) juice to 1/4 cup raw honey and blend well. Take one teaspoon every two hours as needed.

SORE THROAT SYRUP—To soothe a mild sore throat, blend together 1/4 cup raw honey, 1/4 cup glycerine, 1/4 cup of lemon juice, and 2 tablespoons powdered ginger. Place the mixture in a

Sugar / 49

glass jar and immerse the jar in barely boiling hot water. Stir the mixture to blend well. Take one tablespoon as needed.

GRANDMOTHER'S DIARRHEA CURE—Simmer 1/4 cup barley in 10 ounces of water for 20 minutes. Strain and add 2 tablespoons honey while the mixture is still hot. Stir well to dissolve the honey. Sip the entire mixture.

AID FOR THE INSOMNIAC—Steep 1 tablespoon of fresh or dried chamomile in 6 ounces of freshly boiled water. You may add a bit of mint for a refreshing flavor if you like. Stir in a tablespoon of raw honey and sip hot before going to bed.

GRANDMOTHER'S HONEY OINTMENT—Blend together equal parts of sifted flour and raw honey to make a paste. Smooth on skin rashes or simple dermatitis for instant soothing. This is also a well-known aid for a troubled complexion.

COOKING WITH HONEY—To convert a recipe calling for sugar to honey, use 1 cup raw honey plus 1/4 teaspoon of baking soda in place of 1 cup sugar. When baking with honey, keep a close watch. Honey browns rapidly.

Note: Infants and youngsters under one year of age should not be given honey. Their developing digestive systems do not handle it well. Cases of botulism and even death have been reported in tiny tots given honey.

What's The Answer?

If you don't know the answer by now, you haven't been paying attention. The bottom line is that the consumption of sugar (and refined carbohydrates) is one of the major health hazards facing the world today. And switching to NutraSweet, currently the most popular chemical sweetener on the market, may open up another whole can of worms.

Use raw honey in place of sugar. Forget commercially processed sweets loaded with sucrose. Take a few minutes to read the ingredient panel on processed foods. You're in for a big surprise. It's going to be harder than you might think to continue using convenience foods if you decide to take sugar out of your diet.

Supermarkets across the U.S. are full of fresh fruits and vegetables, a prime source of the complex carbohydrates the body needs, at just about any season of the year. It's easy to shop wisely when you're informed. Enjoy the rich and delicious bounty that America offers and find out how it feels to be really healthy.

Great-Grandmother was Right about
Garlic

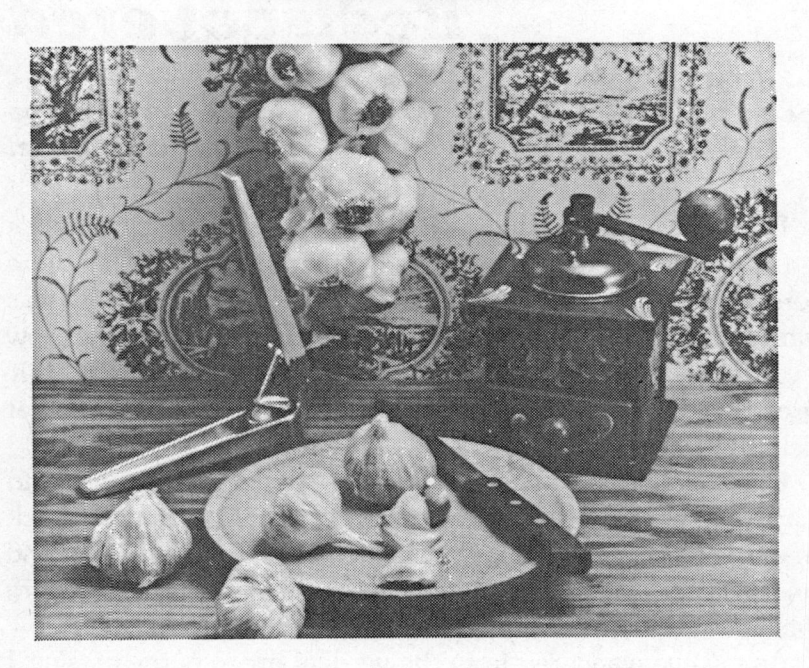

Modern science confirms that garlic is antiseptic, antibacterial, antifungal and bacteriostatic. Garlic, used by healers in over 5,000 years of recorded history, is effective against bronchial congestion, circulatory problems, heart disease and more — and may yet prove to be the cancer-preventive researchers all over the world have been searching for!

CHAPTER 5

Folk Remedy Rediscovered

Science Finds Garlic a Possible Cancer Preventive and More!

Deep in Germany's fabled Black Forest you come with surprise on a huge creaking old farmhouse that looks like it's been there forever, run down now, but still as friendly and welcoming as it was when I was a boy. The farm acreage has turned into a meadow overrun with parsley gone wild, as tall as my knee, the crisp curly green fronds swaying in the breeze very much like a green wheat field run riot.

On vacation last year, I trekked the old paths back to Grandfather and Grandmother's farm and was transported back in memory to green springs and golden summers when my grand and very important doctor father stayed behind in Heidelberg while mother and I summered at the farm.

As my eye wandered from the verdant green of the parsley, I saw the faint outline of Grandmother's kitchen garden and I was suddenly reminded of Brigetta, the hired girl. Brigetta was as hearty and healthy and happy and strong as the milk-cows she tended. She sang at the top of her voice and never minded having me skipping along at her heels. She told me with superstitious awe the legends of the Bavarian country folk — and she smelled as ripe as an old shoe from the cut clove of garlic she wore suspended on a string aroung her neck and the pungent breath she exhaled with gusto. The garlic, she promised me, would keep off the evil eye.

Grandmother, too, was a believer in the power of garlic. Not to ward off the evil eye, but as a medicament and health-protecting food. Every spring, without fail, the first sweet new butter coming from her cows eating the new shoots of grass was turned into her version of a "spring tonic".

As Brigetta churned the butter into nuggets, Grandmother took down a couple of bulbs of dried garlic from the braided string hanging near the kitchen fireplace and pounded them into a mash with her largest pestle in a big worn woooden bowl. When Grandmother had a smooth paste and the fumes were stinging all eyes, Brigetta scooped up a slab of the pale sweet butter and added it to the pounded garlic as Grandmother mixed it in.

When she was satisfied the garlic had permeated every smidgen of the butter, Grandmother then smoothed the aromatic mixture into a heavy crock and lowered it inside a larger crock with many pebbles in the bottom. Brigetta brought in icy-cold water from the well and poured it into the space around the smaller crock and popped on the heavy lid. The crock was kept in the cold-room in the earthen cellar and this primitive ice-chest kept the pungent mixture fresh all summer long.

Although my mother protested, Grandmother insisted, and even mother took a small tangy spoonful after noon supper every day, as we all did. I grew to relish the taste, but Mother rinsed her mouth with salt water and delicately chewed parsley to cleanse and sweeten her breath after downing her portion with an expression of distaste.

Grandmother maintained her pungent garlic paste was an aid to digestion and a sure way to stop a body from succumbing to the coughs, sore throats, colds and sniffles that were a part of life in our frigid winters. Although my scientific-minded father scoffed at such an old remedy, even he became convinced of the great benefits of this herb and became a strong advocate in later years. Thanks to Grandmother's garlic paste, I can testify I was always singularly free of any type of illness or respiratory distress throughout my childhood and sported outside all winter long in the chill air while many of my schoolboy friends sniffled and snuffled and were kept in by their anxious mothers.

Smiling at the thought of the little boy I had been and remembering that Grandfather died at 101 and Grandmother at an incredible 105, I determined to do a little research when I got home to find out if garlic does possess any of the powers Grandmother and Brigetta attributed to that singularly aromatic herb. Like so many other so-called "old-wives tales", I found there is a strong scientific basis for Grandmother's belief. It is very likely my grandparents owed the robust good health they enjoyed well past the Biblical "three-score years and ten" to their daily ration of garlic paste. Garlic *can* protect our health and assists in the cure of many and varied complaints as well.

Garlic Through The Ages & Around the World

In 3748 B.C., Egyptian slaves working on the great pyramid of the Pharoah Cheops staged what was certainly the first sit-down strike in recorded history. Why? The slave-masters stopped their daily ration of garlic! This ancient herb was so highly regarded for its strengthening properties that the slaves risked death rather than be without it.

Ancient Vikings and Phoenicians never set their sails without a healthy supply of garlic on board—and probably avoided coming down with scurvy because of it. Early Chinese, Greeks and Romans used garlic to expel intestinal worms, a common and dangerous complaint of the times, relieve indigestion, heal skin rashes, treat respiratory problems and to stop infection in its tracks. In addition, garlic is thought by many to slow the aging process. In Bulgaria, even today, garlic is still chewed religiously by the general population—and many Bulgarians live active lives past 100-years of age.

Marco Polo, certainly one of the best-known explorers of medieval times and a very prolific and expressive writer, recorded his experience in 13th century Cathay (China) for posterity. In his journal, Marco Polo noted that the higher castes of China ate meat preserved in several expensive special spices—but the poor had to be content with meat steeped in garlic juices! Knowing what we know today, we must conclude the poorer classes had the better of it.

In very early recorded history, the most notable uses of spices and herbs were in medicines, in holy oils, in unguents and as aphrodisiacs. Priests of many sects employed spices and herbs in incantations, rites and ritual worship. Difficult as it may be to believe, garlic was included in this distinguished company. Both the common bulb vegetables, garlic and onions, are pictured on many Egyptian monuments surviving the Pharaohs and are mentioned in many medieval sacred writings as well.

Lloyd J. Harris, in researching garlic, found the decadent Roman aristocracy used garlic because of its power to remove sexual inhibitions and maximize pleasure in sexual activity. Ancient rabbis decreed garlic should be eaten on the night of the Sabbath, the time devoted to marital enjoyment. Certain sex-abstaining religions prohibited the eating of garlic altogether because of the physical desire it creates.

A favored aphrodisiac found in centuries-old Hindu writings, currently enjoying a revival today, is the unlikely combination of garlic and roses! Proponents say this "magic potion" will increase sexual desire and performance, fade wrinkles to make you look years younger and melt away ugly fat bulges. To make the Garlic/Rose Elixir, peel one entire head of garlic and place all cloves (slightly crushed) in a large jar. Add raw natural honey (not the filtered supermarket variety), to cover. Next, take two handfuls of fresh-picked rose petals and crush them. Place the crushed rose petals in a teapot and fill with boiling water. Allow the petals to steep for ten minutes. Add the hot rose petal tea to the garlic-honey mixture slowly and stir gently to melt the honey. Permit the mixture to remain undisturbed for 48 hours for full potency.

Directions for use of this triple-treat "magic potion" are: To banish wrinkles, dilute three tablespoons of the Elixir with a little water and smooth on your face. Leave on for 20 minutes and rinse off with warm water. As a weight-loss appetite depressant, take one tablespoon (undiluted) immediately before eating. To heighten sexual pleasure, both partners should take one tablespoon of the potion (undiluted) immediately before indulging in sexual activity. Experts theorize that it is the phosphorus content of garlic which affects sexual excitability, causing instantaneous and prolonged arousal.

As a medicament, in 1897, master-herbalist W.T. Fernie wrote these words about garlic in his "Herbal Simples," an authoritative healing source of the day, "The bulb, consisting of several cloves, is stimulating, antispasmodic, an expectorant and diuretic. Garlic proves useful in treating asthma, whooping cough and other spasmodic afflictions of the chest, the pain of rheumatic parts may be much relieved by simply rubbing them with cut garlic."

Additional medicinal uses for garlic down through the ages have included tightening loose teeth, removing tartar deposits and the treatment of polio, tuberculosis, ear infections, open wounds, typhus, cholera - and even the Black Plague!

One tale told concerning garlic's amazing powers is purported to have happened during the Great Plague of France. Occurring in 1721, this plague was even more devastasting than the better-known Plague of London. With so many people falling victim to this dreaded disease, it was very difficult to muster the necessary burial details. In desperation, the French government released four condemned convicts from prison and forced them to collect and bury the diseased and highly infectious corpses.

Incredibly, the four condemned thieves appeared to be magically immune to the plague in spite of their close contact with infected bodies in various stages of decay. When the plague had finally run its awful course, the four thieves were promised their freedom if they would reveal the "magic" they used to remain healthy when all around them were dying of the Black Death.

According to the legend, the "magic" potion the condemned men drank daily was a generous portion of sour wine - well steeped with fresh-crushed garlic cloves! This mixture has become known as "Vinaigre des Quatre Voleurs" - Four Thieves Vinegar - and is still sold in France Today!

Just what is this "magic" herb? The Encyclopedia Britannica tells us that garlic (Allium Sativum) is a bulbous perennnial plant of the lily family and is used to flavor foods. The aroma is powerful and onion-like and the taste is pungent. Garlic is a classic ingredient of many national cuisines and has only become popular in the United States since World War II. The bulb contains an antibiotic, *allicin*. Garlic has antiseptic properties and is an expectorant and intestinal antispasmodic.

Garlic is a native vegetable of Central Asia, an area of the world which includes northwest India, Afghanistan and parts of the U.S.S.R. and it grows wild in Italy and southern France. Other vegetables native to the region are carrots, muskmelon, onions, peas, radishes and spinach. Garlic is also indigenous to the Mediterranean, along with artichokes, asparagus, cabbage, celery, chickory, chives, cress, endive, beets, leeks, lettuce, onions, parsley, parsnips, peas, rhubarb and turnips.

The membranous skin of the bulb encloses up to twenty edible bulblets called cloves. Flower stalks sometimes arise bearing tiny bulblets and blossoms without seeds. Garlic is grown as an annual crop by methods similiar to those used in growing onions. Garlic contains about 0.1% essential oil.

Garlic may have arrived on American shores by a circuitous route, but it has a lot of enthusiastic fans. "The Garlic Capital of the World," Gilroy, California (pop. 22,000), annually hosts a fun-filled festival dedicated to garlic. In July of 1984, more than 150,000 garlic fanciers attended!

Scientific Studies Prove Garlic A Superior Natural Remedy

Science says both grandmother and the ancients were right. Among the traditional uses for garlic as a cure are such ailments as asthma, deafness, bronchial congestion, arteriosclerosis, fever, nightmares, circulatory problems and liver conditions. Today, science is not only substantiating the effectiveness of garlic as a remedy for these ills, but is uncovering more and more therapeutic uses for this odiferous herb as well.

Garlic protects against blood clots forming in the veins and its documented anti-clotting agents can help prevent heart attacks and strokes. American scientists have been successful in identifying a chemical, *ajoene*, in garlic which possesses amazing anti-clotting properties. Another chemical with the ability to inhibit the formation of potentially dangerous blood clots is *adenosine*, also present in garlic according to Dr. Martyn Baily of George Washington University, Washington, D.C.

Garlic is both antiseptic and antibacterial. In fact, as long ago as 1858, Louis Pasteur, developer of the pasteurization process that protects our milk from bacterial contamination, reported on the antiseptic powers of garlic. Garlic shows anti-tumor activity and appears to have a tendency to inhibit malignant cells. Current research shows garlic, as a general fungicide, may actually improve the body's all-important immune responses.

Nutritionally speaking, a clove of garlic is an excellent source of potassium and phosphorus. It also contains significant amounts of Vitamins B and C, as well as calcium and protein. And garlic is rich in selenium, currently being studied as a possible heart-disease preventive itself. In addition, selenium is an antioxidant which is said to prevent the effects of aging. Selenium is probably 10 times stronger than Vitamin E and is especially effective in removing contamination by the heavy metals, such as lead and mercury, that enter our bodies through the food chain and the environmental pollution of the air and water supplies of much of the world.

In the laboratories of the world, medical researchers have found garlic to be an amazing natural remedy for many modern ills, including heart-disease, hypertension (high blood pressure), diabetes, dysentery, pneumonia, Candida albicans (fungal/yeast infection) and many others. This wide-acting natural fungicide and antibiotic purifies the blood in the body, removes toxic substances from the cells (by chelation), improves the body's immune system, is a metabolic aid and helps keep weight levels down. Garlic encourages the secretion of hormones within the body, prevents fatigue, promotes the building of energy and helps retain vital B vitamins in the system.

HEALTH INSURANCE FOR THE HEART—In 1971, the University of Michigan mounted a study to discover if eating garlic's pungent oil in capsule form can reduce cholesterol levels in the body. Cholesterol is considered to be a major contributor to heart-disease when it builds up in fatty deposits on artery walls and reduces the flow of blood to the heart.

Two of the university researchers, Alan Tsai, Ph.D., and James Kelley, discovered that when rats were fed a diet moderately high in cholesterol, but which also included garlic, the cholesterol levels rose slightly, but stayed close to normal. Other rats fed the same diet, but without the addition of garlic, showed a skyrocketing 23% increase in their cholesterol levels.

Dr. Hans Reuter, of Cologne, West Germany, found that garlic not only effectively controls cholesterol levels in the blood, but also removes toxins that interfere with the body's metabolism, including the fat-burning process.

Also in 1981, biochemist Amar Makheja, Ph.D., of the George Washington University School of Medicine in Washington D.C., studied garlic's ability to prevent blood clots and subsequent heart attacks. Dr. Makheja says, "The three active ingredients in garlic are adenosine, allicin and a sulphur compound. It's possible that the sulfur compound blocks thromboxane (a clotting agent) and that may be the reason garlic can prevent coronary thrombosis." Dr. Makheja says a regular consumption of garlic is necessary to continue the anti-clotting effect in the blood.

A 1975 study published by Philadelphia's respected Wistar Institute of Anatomy and Biology showed that in rabbits fed a special diet designed to bring on atherosclerosis (hardening and clogging of the arteries), garlic oil reduced cholesterol levels by about 10%. Even better news was the fact that the average fatty deposit on the inner walls of the blood vessels was between 15% and an astounding 45% *less severe* in rabbits fed garlic oil.

These near-miraculous results were confirmed by the Department of Pathology of the R.N.T. Medical College in Udaipur, India where researchers found rabbits who received high cholesterol diets *with garlic oil* were protected to a significant extent. Their arteries were less pitted, showed less evidence of thickening and clogging, and their livers showed only a mild degree of fatty infiltration. Even more exciting was the fact that there was no evidence of cholesterol deposits in the hearts of the rabbits fed garlic oil.

Another Indian study, this time involving humans, was made at the Department of Pharmacology and Medicine, S.N. Medical College, Agra, India. Fed a diet especially prepared to elevate cholesterol levels, ten healthy volunteers ate a high-fat meal. After four hours, cholesterol levels were tested and found almost dangerously high. However, when the same high-fat meal was consumed with garlic, either raw or cooked, cholesterol levels stayed within the low-normal range.

THE CANCER CONNECTION—Wayne E. Criss Ph.D., of Howard's School of Human Ecology, Washington D.C., discovered in a series of experiments done in 1982 that cancers can't grow or spread without a substance called cyclic Guanosine Monophosphate, or cGMP. Dr. Criss then found that an extract from certain plants prevents the formation of cGMP in test tubes. The strongest source of this extract was—you guessed it—garlic!

An early study, published in 1957, continues to inspire scientists to study the effect of garlic on cancer. It was conducted at Case Western Reserve University in Cleveland, Ohio. The chief researcher thought rapidly dividing tissue, including cancer cells, required large amounts of sulfur amino acids. His idea was to cut down on -SH compounds to starve the cancer — and he suspected the active ingredient in garlic, *allicin,* would render the -SH harmless. He decided to find out in a hurry.

Could garlic prevent cancer in mice that had been injected with five million tumor cells that, under ordinary circumstances, would kill them within sixteen days? Producing allicin as nature does, the doctor crushed garlic cloves for his extract. He found that if the allicin was mixed with the tumor cells before the cells were placed in the mice, they didn't get cancer and they didn't die. Not after 16 days—and not after 6 months.

It was the promise shown by this study that encouraged a Japanese effort in 1964. Researchers Yanagi Kimura and Kotaro Yamamoto transplanted live cancer cells into a group of albino rats and injected them with a garlic extract four days later. Within only one hour, the extract produced a marked damage to the tumor cells by blocking the metaphase (a part of the rapid cell-division that characterizes cancer) and by preventing chromosomes from reproducing. Even twelve hours after injection, the garlic extract was still working, fighting about half of the tumor cells, The researchers reported that the tumors shrank, still a near-miraculous effect, but didn't disappear completely.

Three years later, two other Japanese scientists used garlic to develop a sort of "anti-cancer vaccine." As in the earlier American study, they found tumor cells mixed with garlic extract did not produce a cancer in mice. Carrying their experiments further, they found an injection of garlic-saturated tumor cells actually immunized the mice against at least one type of cancer.

The two researchers twice injected mice with the "anti-cancer vaccine" of live tumor cells soaked in garlic extract, giving the shots one week apart. When the mice were then injected with cancer cells fourteen days after immunization, none developed tumors and none died within a time period of 100 days when the experiment was ended. By comparison, mice injected with live tumor cells *without the vaccine* died within just 14 to 28 days.

Dr. Mei Xing of the Shandong Medical College believes his 1981 study of cancer rates in China shows that the regular consumption of garlic results in a lower rate of stomach cancer. Dr. Xing says garlic juices seem to inhibit the growth of bacteria in the stomach, with less formation of nitrites and nitrosamines. Nitrosamines are known to cause cancer in animals. In an experiment, he found that volunteers who took 1/3 ounce of homogenized fresh garlic reduced their nitrite levels significantly within only four hours. Dr. Xing says, "Garlic reduces the concentration of nitrite in the human stomach and may thus be considered as a protective factor against the development of gastric (stomach) cancer."

TRIPLE PROTECTION: ANTIBIOTIC, ANTIFUNGAL & BACTERIOSTATIC PROPERTIES—In testing antibiotics against various infections, clinical microbiologist Edward Delaha of Georgetown University Hospital of Washington, D.C. found garlic often works as well as chemically-manufactured antibiotics. Delaha says a shampoo of powdered garlic and chlorophyll might cure scalp infections, such as ringworm, and athlete's foot could be eliminated by a simple soaking in garlic water.

Delaha says, "Garlic seems to be extremely effective. They've been using injections of garlic extract on patients with a type of meningitis caused by a fungus in China. They've had an unbelievable cure rate, even with people who have been in comas."

YEAST INFECTIONS—The medical treatment of choice for fungal infections is the use of antifungal drugs. However, the side-effects of these prescribed drugs include the possibility of kidney damage, nausea, fever, skin rashes and so on. Science now recognizes that Candida albicans, considered by many to be merely the vaginitis that plagues so many women, is actually a serious threat to health and can escalate into many more diseases, including meningitis and encephalitis. It is not limited to women only and typically attacks those in an already weakend condition from other illnesses.

Recent clinical research has identified Candida albicans as the root cause of many symptoms, such as vaginitis (and a similar condition in the male partner), mouth thrush, tiredness, depression and even "bad moods." The symptoms of Candida can be manifested in anything from allergies and eye infections to an inflammation of the colon.

Fortunately, garlic is non-toxic and has been shown to inhibit the growth of fungus in the body without the adverse side-effects of drugs. The active component of garlic is stable in both the blood and stomach and acts effectively in the body's acidic environment.

The antibiotic, antifungal and bacteriostatic effects of garlic come from *allicin*, formed when the cellular membrane of the garlic clove is sliced or crushed. The cellular membrane separates an enzyme, *allinase*, and the substrate *alliin*. Mixed together, they create *allicin*—and the characteristic odor associated with this pungent herb. But it's the allicin we want. Allicin has the wonderful ability to attack harmful bacteria within the body without attacking and destroying the beneficial bacteria and digestive flora we need. In fact, some researchers have noted allicin can be more effective and is often needed in smaller quantities than penicillin.

Garlic has been called "Russian penicillin," probably because it was widely used by U.S.S.R. doctors to treat the wounded during two world wars. A cut clove of garlic was placed around infected wounds and held in place with a light bandage. Incredibly, within a few days, the wound was completely clean with no sign of infection or putrid flesh. Currently, U.S.S.R. scientists have discovered a method of reducing garlic to a vapor and this vapor is then inhaled. Unfortunately, I have been unable to turn up any concrete information as to the results of such a highly novel garlic treatment. It seems to me much easier just to add garlic to the daily diet in one form or another.

HIGH BLOOD PRESSURE—As long ago as 1948, a Dr. Piotrowski of the University of Geneva, publishing in the medical journal *PRAXIS*, reported on experiments he conducted with a group of 100 patients suffering from hypertension, or high blood pressure.

His research revealed that within three to five days of garlic treatment, over 40% of these patients had a satisfactory reduction in their blood pressure.

BLOOD SUGAR REDUCED IN DIABETICS—In a 1973 edition of *LANCET*, three doctors published reports showing that garlic was equally as effective as the drug tolbutamide, medical treatment of choice in the management of diabetes. The three doctors, working independently, all established that garlic, slower acting than the drug tolbutamide, could actually clear the blood stream of excessive glucose.

GARLIC AGAINST COLDS, COUGHS, BRONCHITIS, ASTHMA—A medical practitioner by the name of K. Nolfi, M.D. author of *"My Experiences with Living Food,"* writes that garlic is effective against all manner of respiratory infections. Dr. Nolfi's method of curing the common cold consists of holding a cut clove of garlic inside the mouth between the cheeks and teeth. It is said this method will cure a cold almost immediately. For more serious complaints, including badly inflamed tonsils and glands, laryngitis and bronchitis, the cut cloves of garlic must be renewed every few hours over a period of a few days. Dr. Nolfi also says a cut clove of garlic rubbed on the soles of the feet before retiring will often cure a cold overnight, but didn't explain how to avoid chasing your bed partner out of the room in the process!

As you can see from the studies reported on, the serious research on garlic's properties is currently centered on the effect this pungent herb has against the two biggest killers of modern times—cancer and heart-disease. Although the encouraging results being shown by scientists around the world are hard to believe in this chemically oriented and prescription drug age we live in, all are true and well-documented. This common herb, shunned by many sophisticated people because it causes "garlic-breath," has been proven of great value in over 5,000 years of recorded use, as well as in the laboratories of today.

Many Forms Of Garlic On The Market

If you have decided to add garlic to your daily diet, as I have, you will probably want to visit a local health-food store and look over the many forms of garlic preparations currently on the market. When making your selection, make sure the product you select contains the natural *allicin,* the active antibiotic, antifungal and bacteriostatic component of raw garlic. Some manufacturers have taken out the allicin in order to produce an odorless garlic.

However, at least one responsible manufacturer, the Wakunaga Pharmaceutical Company of Japan, produces and distributes a deodorized garlic in tablets, capsules and liquid under the trademark *Kyolic®*. All Kyolic garlic products contain a modified form of allicin the company claims to be better than the real thing. As a chelating agent, Kyolic is said to exert a detoxifying effect which neutralizes heavy metal poisoning by binding with lead, mercury and cadmium and acts as an antioxidant as well, thus improving the function of the liver, kidneys, nervous system and circulatory system.

In addition to a liquid garlic extract, you will find other odorless forms still containing allicin, but specially processed to prevent any hint of garlic from tainting your breath. You might choose a garlic/parsely combination in either tablets or capsules, or even a potent 1000 mg garlic capsule with 2 mgs of nature's breath sweetener, chlorophyll.

If you decide on a capsule, I want to add one word of caution here, and this goes for any food product you purchase as well. *Be sure the product you choose is not made with hydrogenated oil of any type.* This is an all too common ingredient in many processed foods. Doesn't sound threatening, does it? In fact, however, hydrogenated oil is extremely harmful to the body.

All natural fats and oils contain substances known as *antioxidants,* which prevent rancidity. When allowed to remain in foods, these *antioxidants prevent the destruction of Vitamins A, D, E, K, several B Vitamins and carotene—not only in food itself, but in the intestinal tract.* Without natural antioxidants, serious losses of these vitamins occur before they can reach the blood.

Unfortunately, the natural antioxidants are lost when fats and oils are hydrogenated. Hydrogen is added to the unfilled chain of essential fatty acids, destroying their health-building value. Untreated, unrefined cold-pressed oils still contain most of their antioxidants and can be purchased at most health-food stores.

Among all the forms of garlic now available, we bring to your attention here a new biologically active garlic preparation called *Garlisan*™ (garlic heals) we have discovered which was just released in 1986. Using the very latest in space-age technology, garlic cloves are harvested and processed straight from the garden to capture and preserve all the volatile oils and natural elements. The end result is a capsule containing all the vital health-promoting activity of this pungent herb. Studies comparing this method of processing with freshly harvested garlic show that the active constituents in both are one and the same.

Garlisan, a new and unique capsulized form of garlic, also contains *alfalfa* and *capsicum* (cayenne), an exclusive formulation which synergistically potentiates the scientifically documented healthful properties of the garlic itself.

Alfalfa (Medicago sativa) not only contains chlorophyll, nature's deodorizer and breath freshener, but is rich in essential nutrients, vitamins (A, D, K), digestive enzymes, and important minerals (calcium, phosphorus, iron, potassium). Alfalfa is a noted germicide, and helps break down carbon dioxide in the system. Because it is mildly diuretic, it assists the body in eliminating excess fluids, thereby relieving urinary and bowel distress

Alfalfa has been used for centuries as a tonic, nervine, and kidney cleanser. Herbalists and nutritionists alike praise the amazing health building properties of alfalfa.

Capsicum (Capsicum frutescens or Capsicum minimum), better known as cayenne, acts as a catalyst for all other herbs. It has the incredible ability to quickly carry other ingredients to the parts of the body where they are most needed, both stimulating and increasing the effectiveness of any remedy. Capsicum is useful in relieving all types of congestion. Because it acts to reduce engorged and dilated blood vessels (thereby assisting heart action and stimulating the circulation of healthy oxygenated blood), capsicum is said to aid in preventing strokes, heart attacks, and internal hemorrhaging.

Capsicum offers the Vitamins A, B-Complex, C, and G. It is rich in potassium, iron and calcium, plus certain vital trace minerals (magnesium, phosphorus, and sulphur). Because it assists the immune system, capsicum is considered a good natural stimulant which builds and promotes health and wards off disease.

This technologically superior form of garlic should be available in health food stores nationwide very soon. If you have difficulty locating *Garlisan*, call 1-800-624-7114 (Extension 18) toll-free for information on ordering by mail.

If you fancy fresh garlic, but don't want to offend others with the pungency of your breath, one recommended method is to finely mince a portion of a clove, put it in a teaspoon and place it on the back of your tongue. Swallow quickly with a glass of water. Chewing is what releases garlic's characteristic odor and causes it to scent—or foul—the breath, depending on your point of view!

One husband and wife I know of have solved the breath problem in still another way. Neither wishes to offend the other, but both believe very strongly in the health-promoting and preventive effects of fresh garlic. Here's what they do. Just before retiring, the wife chops a fresh cut clove of garlic into small pieces. Then she peels a banana, slits it down the middle and tucks the garlic inside. Both husband and wife eat their half-banana laced with garlic and they go to bed. They report there is absolutely no odor of garlic on the breath, not even the next morning!

Whatever your choice, remember garlic is highly effective as a natural preventive and should be taken daily for best results.

CHAPTER 6

The Miracle of Linseed Oil

The Medicinal Fat

A very good friend, George Friedrich, suffered three serious heart attacks between the ages of sixty and sixty-three. At the rate of one heart attack every year, his doctors didn't hold out much hope for a complete recovery. George's entire cardiovascular system was clogged with atherosclerotic plaque, interrupting the vital blood flow to his heart. He was put on very strong medicine, including nitroglycerin for his angina pain, and was taking up to fifteen pills every day.

During the three years of his early sixties, George became very weak and aged visibly. He was on a downhill course until he was introduced to *Dr. Johanna Budwig's Formula*. He immediately incorporated Dr. Budwig's Formula into his daily diet. For breakfast every morning, he took 1 tablespoon of cold-processed unrefined linseed oil mixed with low-fat cottage cheese. In order to make this fare more palatable, he added different herbs, raw vegetables, or fruits for variety. George found his favorite additions were a mixture of finely grated cucumbers and radishes with finely chopped tomatoes.

After eating this low-fat cottage cheese 'salad' daily for just three months, George found his breathing was easing and the angina pain that had been with him for so long was almost eliminated. A year later, the medical doctors who examined him were amazed at his full recovery. Even his tiniest capillaries were as clean as those of a much younger man. Today, at sixty-five, George no longer needs any pills. Needless to say, he is very grateful to have discovered Dr. Budwig's Formula in time.

Who Is Dr. Johanna Budwig?

Dr. Johanna Budwig, a well-known and highly respected German biochemist, has published her research on the properties and benefits of linseed oil under the title *True Health Against Arteriosclerosis, Heart Infarction, & Cancer*. Although Dr. Budwig is not a practicing physician, she has assisted many seriously ill individuals, even those given up as terminal by orthodox medical practitioners, to regain their health through a simple regimen of nutrition. The basis of Dr. Budwig's program is the use of linseed oil blended with cottage cheese.

Because her research has been highly publicized in Europe, even the man on the street has long been aware of the dangers of consuming too much of the wrong kind of fat. To illustrate this point, Dr. Budwig tells a charming story published in the London Daily Express headlined *"Fat In Your Frying Pan Can Kill."*

A husband returning home from an exhausting day at work said to his wife, "Pan fry me a steak, dear, but throw the fat away." "Certainly, not!" replied his wife. "The fat I'll use to crisp your steak the way you like it cost 36 cents! Do you really want me to throw away 36 cents?" The husband, in mock horror, answered, "What! Your husband isn't worth 36 cents to you?"

Dr. Budwig teaches that the way in which the body metabolizes fat concerns every vital organ in the body, pointing out that people afflicted with liver and gallbladder problems in particular cannot tolerate fat. She also observes that a high-fat diet dosen't agree with any unhealthy person, but explains that the three-times unsaturated, oxygenated fats in linseed oil, when taken with protein-rich cottage cheese, are easily tolerated by anyone, even those seriously ill.

Dr. Budwig tells of giving a lecture in Switzerland to hundreds of people. As she was taking questions from the audience, a man and wife approached the podium and asked to tell the listeners of their experiences. Dr. Budwig passed the man the microphone and, with tears in his eyes, he began to speak. He told of his daughter who had serious deterioration of one knee joint. Her doctors had said her condition was incurable, that medical science had no hope for her, that she would eventually be completely bedridden and, unable to care for herself, would require full-time nursing care in a sanitorium. The unfortunate young girl also suffered from a disfiguring case of psoriasis. The man said that he himself had a tumor in one lung and went on to tell of the health problems of his son. When the man was overcome by emotion, his wife took the microphone and completed the story. She said that when she began insisting the entire family follow Dr. Budwig's recommendation to eat linseed oil with cottage cheese every day, gradually their health improved. She reported that all four members of the family regained complete and robust health on Dr. Budwig's simple regimen.

Dr. Johanna Budwig Speaks

Dr. Budwig lectures all over Europe. Her fame precedes her and she is acclaimed on the continent for her important work. Thousands flock to hear her speak whenever she appears. The many people she has helped revere her and testify to the benefits of her simple program of health. In order to bring you news of Dr. Budwig's revolutionary approach to the cure and treatment of cancer, heart infarction, arteriosclerosis, and stroke in her own words, we have had a wealth of her printed material translated into the English language and excerpt as follows:

"As far back as 1957, the Cancer Research Institute of Paris, France began studies to determine the exact difference between a cancer cell and a normal cell. As revealed during the International Congress of Nutrition, the French scientists announced that they had found a lot of undissolved fat deposited in the nucleus, body and plasma of the cancer cell. In his book, *The Cancer Problem,* Professor Bauer of Germany said that fat can both dissolve tumors and cause tumors. Although at the time this statement appeared contradictory, we know now that there are many different types of fat.

"Following this line of reasoning, it is obvious that if we feed the body the highly unsaturated and oxygenated essential fatty acids it requires, along with the high quality protein which makes fat easily soluble, it will counteract toxic and poisonous accumulations in the tissues. If we also stay away from chemical preservatives, then many, many people will become healthy very fast—even some who have been given up by doctors and hospitalized to die. I have proved this premise many times.

"Every part of the body is affected adversely by the use of saturated fats, including the brain, the liver, the kidneys, and the nervous system. But the function of the heart is perhaps the hardest hit when a disturbance in the fat metabolism occurs. When the wrong kind of fat has been ingested, it is transported via the blood lymph. Fat globules (atherosclerotic plaque) are deposited in these vital pathways leading to heart disease.

"Poor nutrition gives rise to many problems. For instance, I once visited a woman in Switzerland who was suffering from terminal cancer. As a mother, her main concern was not herself, but the health of her two children, a boy 12 and a girl 14. Both were obese and looked ill. I gathered the little family together and spoke to them of the importance of eating correctly. The daughter said to me in a soft voice, "What is this wonderful preparation that can make us all well?" I explained how to prepare a cottage cheese salad dressed with linseed oil and how it could benefit the entire household.

"On the whole, I blame the older generation for the generally poor health of so many. Foods are commonly over processed and chemical additives are used to extend the shelf life and make more money for the manufacturers. The wrong kinds of fats are used and they are not pure. Many sexual dysfunctions are caused because the body cannot metabolize these foods. Fortunately, many health problems can be easily remedied simply by correcting the diet.

"When I talk about my linseed oil/high-quality protein fare, it is nothing but a simple food which contains the most active fat known to me: linseed oil. In this form, the essential fatty acids are easily assimilated and made soluble in connection with essential amino acids (protein) in the form of cottage cheese. This is good tasting and very palatable. It has been used in Europe for many years by hundreds of thousands of individuals.

"I tell you now that this simple food can inhibit the growth of tumors. By completely natural means, fat metabolism is stimulated and the size of the tumor actually decreases. Of course, it is better that you not wait until three or four doctors and several hospitals have told you that your tumor is incurable. Instead, regain maximum health by always using the best nutrition. In a very short period of time, even the most seriously ill person will feel better.

"Very often I go into hospitals and take home very seriously sick cancer patients who have been told they don't have long to live. The first improvement which encourages these sick people and their families is when they say things like: "In the hospital, I couldn't urinate." "In the hospital, I couldn't have a bowel movement." "In the hospital, I couldn't clear the mucus from my throat." Suddenly all those blockages clear and the system becomes activated again simply because the linseed oil and cottage cheese I give are rich in essential fatty acids and electrons which emulsify the blockages and remove them. Sick people tell me, "I feel so much lighter and not dragged down and heavy any more."

"We have to return to this immune biological way of eating. I have been to Japan, China, and even India attending many scientifically oriented symposiums and have connections with many researchers in this field. They all wonder the same thing: "Why is it that the biological approach of treating disease is so often attacked by authorities in the orthodox medical field?" I myself have been to court many times to defend my beliefs.

Fortunately, all courts ruled in my favor.

"What is it that I am doing? It's very simple. If any cancer patient comes to me, I just give them simple, natural nutrition. That's all. What can we learn from all this?

"First, we must restore correct nutrition. Fats, proteins, fruits and vegetables are very important. But we have to be careful to take them in an unrefined and totally natural state as nature intended.

"Second, we should be careful to avoid foods which have been contaminated with chemicals through processing or refining or treatment with antibiotics and growth hormones.

"To stay healthy and maintain all the vital functions of the body, we absolutely must be able to metabolize fat efficiently. The continuing research on fat metabolism in connection with oxygenation, absorption, and assimilation of energy is of immense importance. If we are to survive in the western civilized world as a human being and a race, it's time to think about living our lives through sound biological principles.

"The secret of the wisdom of the universe is that science must conform with nature. Science and nature must work in harmony. Time is running out for all of us. We must begin to think and act and, most importantly, *eat responsibly* for the health and welfare of the race."

Linseed—Past & Present

THEN—You might be more familiar with linseed (Linum usitatissimum) as *flax*. Since prehistoric times, this graceful plant with its long, flat, elliptical seeds has been prized for its fibre, from which linen is made, and for the rich oil given up by its seed.

Ayurvedic herbalists recognized the importance of linseed as a medicinal centuries ago. (*Ayurveda* is a very old Hindu system of natural medicine still practiced in some parts of Asia.) Herbologists consider the ripe oil-rich seeds of this botanical a superior internal demulcent (softening agent) and also use them in poultices for the treatment of rheumatism, gout, boils, and carbuncles. The oil is used as an enema to treat impacted feces. Mixed with lime water, the oil can be applied topically to promote the healing of skin lesions and to soothe the intolerable itch of eczema. The bark and leaves are believed to fight venereal diseases, especially gonorrhea.

The ancient Greeks and Romans used the brown, shiny seeds as a natural protein staple in their diet, and their ancestors followed suit as they spread across the entire European continent. The plant grows well in any temperate climate and was known in old India and parts of Russia, as well as South America and the early American colonies.

NOW—Linseed oil continues to be cultivated and is regarded as a high-quality vegetable oil in many parts of the world today, but most Americans look on it as merely an additive in oil-based paints or as livestock feed. In this country, the meal which remains after the oil is removed is compressed into cakes and used as a high-protein mineral-rich livestock food.

The central Europeans, in particular, value the healthful properties of this remarkable plant. Our cousins across the ocean can purchase cold-pressed and *unrefined* raw linseed oil as easily as we can purchase the over-processed, chemicalized and hydrogenated abominations that pass for vegetable oils lining the shelves of our local supermarkets.

THE OIL—Because the linseeds themselves contain from 33 to 43 percent oil, they give up their valuable liquid fat quite easily when compressed. When it hasn't been heated, filtered, and refined, the raw cold-pressed linseed oil is a rich golden-yellow, amber, or brownish liquid. It thickens and becomes more viscous on exposure to air. Note: Unrefined linseed oil retains full potency for approximately three months before losing quality.

The light-colored refined variety which flows almost as easily as water, the only type of linseed oil available to the consumer currently in the U.S. (even in health food stores), has had all the valuable solid fats (the essential fatty acids the body requires) removed. Unfortunately, it cannot be considered an adequate substitute for the linseed oil we are discussing in this chapter.

RAW LINSEED OIL—In its *unrefined* form, linseed oil contains two important unsaturated fatty acids (cis-linoleic and gamma-linoleic). When correctly processed, the oil consists of a healthy 58 percent linoleic acids. These essential highly unsaturated fatty acids are converted in the body to *prostaglandins*.

In Europe, raw linseed oil is used therapeutically in the prevention and treatment of: *(1)* Cancer, *(2)* Arteriosclerosis (reduces arteriosclerotic plaque/cholesterol & tri-glyceride levels), *(3)* Strokes & Cardiac Infarction, *(4)* Heartbeat (irregular), *(5)* Red blood corpuscles (maintains flexibility), *(6)* Liver damage, *(7)* Lungs (reduces bronchial spasms), *(8)* Intestines (regulates activity), *(9)* Stomach Ulcers (normalizes gastric juices), *(10)* Prostate (hypertrophic), *(11)* Arthritis (exerts a favorable influence), *(12)* Eczema (assists all skin disease), *(13)* Old Age (improves many common afflictions), *(14)* Brain (strengthens activity), and *(15)* Immune Deficiency Syndromes (Cancer, Multiple Sclerosis, auto-immune illness).

Without essential fatty acids, prostaglandin biosynthesis cannot take place. The biological importance of prostaglandins lies in their high effectiveness, the range and diversity of their metabolic actions, and their wide distribution in the body. These chemically active substances affect the cardiovascular system, are present in the prostate gland, menstrual fluid, the brain, the lungs, the kidneys, the thymus gland, seminal fluid, and the pancreas. There are more than a dozen extremely important prostaglandins. All are derived from essential fatty acids. Without the essential fatty acids (present and active in raw linseed oil), the body cannot manufacture the prostaglandins it needs for healthy functioning.

Considering the important part essential fatty acids play in manufacturing prostaglandins, it's easy to see why raw linseed oil is so therapeutically important and why the current research coming out of Europe can benefit us all in a preventive approach to many diseases.

World-Wide Research

THE USE OF LINSEED OIL—Linseed oil is an edible polyunsaturated vegetable oil and is used in cooking in many parts of the world. It is very rich in essential polyunsaturated fats (linoleic and linolenic acids). Because these fatty acids are known to be essential to the body, many researchers around the world are investigating their properties and trying to determine the benefits of adding linseed oil to the diet. The results reported by various scientific authorities, excerpted below, are truly astounding.

GREAT BRITAIN—This very interesting study entitled *Changes in the Rumen Metabolism of Sheep Given Increasing Amounts of Linseed Oil in Their Diet* gives an indication of the function of linseed oil and how it can benefit the body.

We quote, "It appears that the lowering of the concentration of acetate in the rumen was not the result of decreased production, but rather increased utilization, such as one would expect if lipid synthesis increased. Linseed oil added to the diet did not depress VFA (volatile fatty acids) production, but actually increased it. Results confirmed that up to 25 grams of additional lipids could be synthesized by supplying linseed oil with the sheeps' diet."

A 'translation' follows. *Acetate* is a substance produced in the body when fats are not properly metabolized. However, when linseed oil was added to their diet, the contents of the sheeps' *rumen* (first stomach) showed that, even on this extremely high-fat feed, the *lipids* (fats) were being efficiently used.

POLAND—In a paper entitled *The Cytotoxic Action of Unsaturated Fatty Acids on Cancer*, the Department of Pharmaceutical Technology of the Medical Academy, Wroclaw, Poland, announced: "The fatty acids isolated from linseed oil were found to exhibit a strong cytotoxic in vitro activity against Ehrlich ascites cancer cells with minimal cytotoxic effect on normal cells (leukocytes) of the peritoneal exudate in rabbits. The fatty acids from linseed oil (1000 g/ml after a 3 hour incubation) gave 100 percent dead carcinoma cells."

In plain English, the near-miraculous news is that the active elements of linseed oil exerted a *cytotoxic* (cell destroying) action against cancer cells *in vitro* (literally, in 'glass,' as in a test tube or lab dish), but bypassed healthy *leukocytes* (white blood cells).

GERMANY—From the Department of Pharmacology & Toxicology, Martin Luther Universtiy in Wittenburg, Germany, comes a research paper entitled *The Influence of a Linseed Oil Diet on Fatty Acid Patterns in Phospholipids & Thromboxane Formation in Platelets in Man.*

Interest in mounting this study developed due to the fact that Greenland Eskimos, who traditionally eat a diet high in EPA (known to increase the metabolism of fat), rarely suffer from heart disease. Building on the work of G. Hornstra (as published in Lancet 1979), the bottom line is that this paper demonstrates that a diet rich in linseed oil can lower the risk of arterial thrombosis.

Noting that "A linseed oil diet is known as a 'prudent diet' in Germany," the scientists reported: "A diet of linseed oil (30 ml daily) for four weeks raised the content of x-linolenic acids by twofold, of EPA (eicosapentaenoic acid) by 150 percent, and of decosahexaenoic acid by 70 percent in the serum of volunteers. The human body seems capable of transforming linolenic acid into EPA. This change coincided with a significantly reduced production of platelet thromboxanes (clotting agents)."

INDIA—The Department of Medicine, Patna Medical College & Hospital, Patna, India, has released the results of a study entitled *Influence of Linseed Oil on Cholesterol-Induced Atherosclerosis in Rabbits.* Begining with the premise that many researchers have shown that saturated fats increase the severity of atherosclerosis, the Indian doctors administered 25 g linseed oil with their feed to 36 albino rabbits for a period of 18 weeks.

At the close of the experiment, the animals were sacrificed and the researchers reported: "Atherosclerotic lesions were absent in group L (fed linseed oil), but the percentage of atherosclerotic lesions was significantly high in the control groups (not given linseed oil)."

It is important to note that in the group of animals given PUFA (polyunsaturated fatty acids) along with a cholesterol-inducing diet of saturated fats, a greater incidence of cholesterol buildup was noted. Of this statistic, the scientists say: "The hypercholesterolemic effect of (the combination of) saturated *and* unsaturated fat in rabbits fed cholesterol is caused by increased absorption and retention of cholesterol."

Does this mean that all polyunsaturated fats are not created equal? Apparently so. Linseed oil itself is a highly polyunsaturated fat, but did not contribute to a buildup of harmful cholesterol or atherosclerotic plaque.

AUSTRALIA—Coming to us from the Royal Perth Hospital of the University of Western Australia 'down under,' is a study entitled *An Inhibitory Effect of Dietary Polyunsaturated Fatty Acids (PUFAs) on Renin Secretion in the Isolated Perfused Rat Kidney*. In case you're confused, slowing down (inhibiting) the production of *renin*, is good. Renin is a protein that masquerades as an enzyme and acts as a powerful *vasoconstrictor* (compressing the veins and restricting the vital free flow of blood).

Excerpting from this paper: "After a four-week regimen of diets enriched with linseed oil, safflower oil, or saturated fat (providing 20 percent of the total daily energy intake), the animals fed linseed oil showed a significant fall in the proportion of arachidonic acids in renal phospholipids (kidney fats) and a reduction in urinary prostaglandin excretion. In comparison with the other dietary groups, linseed oil feeding also resulted in a consistently lower renal vascular tone. Results suggest that dietary enrichment with PUFAs may contribute to the lower blood pressures observed." In theory, it might be said that the superior effects of the linseed oil diet are related to increased vasodilator (vein expansion) activity.

Another study from the same source entitled *Dietary Modification of Platelet & Renal Prostaglandins* provides a clearer explanation of the lowered blood pressure readings observed, as follows: "Changes in renal (kidney) function and blood pressure control were reversed by restoring essential fatty acids to the diet. Dietary linseed oil caused the incorporation of linolenic acid into plasma and kidney lipids with a relatively minor reduction in arachidonic acid when compared to the hydrogenated coconut oil control. Diets rich in linoleic acid have also been shown to delay the onset of hypertension (high blood pressure).

"Prostaglandins are synthesized from arachidonic acid which, in turn, is produced from dietary linoleic acid. Prostaglandins are involved in a number of blood pressure regulating mechanisms and have potent direct vascular effects. Significant changes in fatty acids and prostaglandin metabolism can be achieved with fat supplements of less than 40 percent of energy. Rats on an oil-rich diet showed an average lower blood pressure than animals on the standard diet."

FRANCE—The National Institute of Alimentary Research, Dijon Cedex, France, has published a report entitled *The Transference of Cyclic Monomeric Acids into the Milk of Rats Ingesting Thermopolymerized Linseed Oil*. The result of this study of pregnant and nursing female rats fed linseed oil interjects a cautionary note into the otherwise unblemished record of dietary linseed oil.

The researchers found that the administration of linseed oil (100 g of linseed oil thermopolymerized at 275 degrees centigrade per kilogram of feed) to female rats during the period of gestation and lactation caused the death of all young, either at birth or in the two weeks following birth. Rats on a regular commercial diet up to the day of littering gave birth to normal young. When these same females were given linseed oil in their diet during the nursing period, the young rats did not die, but their rate of growth was measurably slowed.

WARNING—Although the amount of linseed oil fed the female rats in this study was proportionately much greater than would normally be ingested by a pregnant woman supplementing her diet with this nutrient, the results of this important research certainly indicate that *a women who is (or suspects she might be) pregnant should not include linseed oil in her diet until after giving birth and weaning the child.*

AUSTRALIA—The Microbiology Department of the Royal Melbourne Hospital in Victoria, Australia published a paper in 1981 entitled *Antibacterial Activity of Hydrolysed Linseed Oil & Linolenic Acid Against Methicillin-Resistant Staphylococcus Aureus (MSRA).*

We quote: "Methicillin-Resistant strains of Staphylococcus aureus, which are also resistant to most other anti-staphylococcal antibiotics, are currently causing a widespread epidemic of hospital-acquired infection in the State of Victoria. Patients who are colonized with MRSA appear to run a greater risk of infection after operative or other invasive procedures than do those who lack these strains."

"For many strains (of MRSA) at low concentrations of linolenic acid and hydrolysed linseed oil, there was striking reduction in the size of the colonies. Our data show that MRSA are sensitive to hydrolyzed linseed oil as well as linolenic acid. Preparations containing hydrolyzed linseed oil may have a role in the eradication of the staphylococcal carrier state and could also be useful for prophylaxis, especially in debilitated patients."

Not only in Australia, but all over the world, the risk of contracting a staph infection while in a hospital is very real. This landmark report on the antibacterial effects of linseed oil (and linolenic acid) should be given world-wide attention.

Some Heart-Warming Stories

Coming out of Europe, and most especially stemming from the work of German biochemist Dr. Johanna Budwig, we hear astounding reports on the great benefits of simply adding linseed oil to the diet. Dr. Budwig reports that the essential fatty acids present in raw, cold-processed, unrefined linseed oil drizzled over one-half cup of protein-rich cottage cheese (please select the low-fat variety) daily apparently works wonders. Read on.

BASAL CELL CARCINOMA—An elderly woman of 76 years of age, Mrs. Erika H., was afflicted with a somewhat slow-growing cancer on the tip of her nose which nevertheless was developing into a particularly ugly and disfiguring *rodent ulcer*. (A rodent ulcer is a gnawing cancer which eats through soft tissue and bone.) Because of Mrs. H.'s advanced age and the site of the cancer, her physician was understandably reluctant to operate and was attempting to treat her in the traditional manner.

Although Mrs. H. disliked being seen in public, a neighbor persuaded her to attend a lecture given by Dr. Johanna Budwig which was being held in a nearby town. After hearing Dr. Budwig speak, Mrs. H. began taking the linseed oil/cottage cheese combination religiously, adding a few cooking herbs from her kitchen garden to overcome the oily taste. She also applied linseed oil directly to the site of the cancer every evening before retiring. Very slowly, the affected tissue on the tip of her nose began to regenerate and eventually the ulcer healed. Mrs H.'s physician credits modern medical techniques, but Mrs. H. herself believes with all her heart that Dr. Budwig's 'recipe for health' was responsible for her near-miraculous cure.

CARCINOMA OF THE STOMACH—When Mr. William Y. (42 years of age, husband and father of three) began suffering from chronic indigestion, he chalked it up to the stress of his job as a prominent officer of the local bank. He took over-the-counter antacid compounds to relieve his distress and ignored the problem. The condition persisted and his wife began urging him to see a doctor, but he stubbornly refused. He soon began vomiting half-digested food after eating and noticed streaks of blood in his stools after a bowel movement. Frightened and worried by these developments, Mr. Y. visited his doctor who immediately rushed him to the hospital for tests. His worst fears were realized when his doctor informed him that it appeared he had a malignant tumor growing in his digestive tract. Fortunately for Mr. Y., there was as yet no involvement of the lymph glands. (Because the lymph travels swiftly through the body, any involvement of the lymph nodes means that the malignancy can spread very quickly to other sites. In the case of lymph cancer, prognosis is extremely poor.)

Mr. Y underwent an operation to surgically remove (excise) the cancerous growth, which appeared to be totally enclosed within its outer membrane. However, because of the possible danger of the blood stream carrying minute cancer cells to other parts of the body, Mr. Y. was placed on a program of advanced chemotherapy on an out-patient basis. He suffered all the classic side-effects of this toxic treatment, including violent vomiting and retching, progressive physical weakness, and almost complete loss of hair. The exhausted and nauseated Mr. Y. complained that the 'cure' was almost too terrible to bear.

Finally, a sympathetic friend brought Mrs. Y. some printed material which told in detail of the success of linseed oil and enriched protein in cases similar to that of her husband. The desperate wife and mother purchased some cottage cheese and a vial of raw, cold-processed, unrefined linseed oil and coaxed Mr. Y. to have it as his luncheon every day. Beginning by choking down just a few small spoonfuls daily, Mr. Y. progressed to the point where he was able to enjoy the entire amount. At this writing, Mr. Y. has returned to his employment as a bank officer and is once again able to support his family. He has completely regained his former robust health. As a preventive measure, the entire family now takes a salad of linseed oil and cottage cheese flavored with a variety of flavorful herbs daily.

HYPERTENSION—A harried and stressed criminal attorney of 47 years of age, Mr. Whitman W. was not surprised when his physician told him he was suffering from high blood pressure and would have to take prescribed medication for the rest of his life as he was risking collapse from heart attack or stroke. Mr. W.'s doctor also advised him to take a vacation and take it easy in his professional life. Mr. W. laughed shortly and briefly outlined the important cases he had on his calendar that would require long days and longer nights of dedicated hard work and intense concentration. He continued working at his normal furious pace until he was faced with extreme exhaustion and could no longer ignore his health.

Mr. W. was finally forced to turn his case load over to a colleague. He checked into a renowned European health clinic and spa and prepared to take the rest he needed to renew himself. The director of this famous clinic was an advocate of linseed oil and insisted that the patients be served linseed oil and cottage cheese daily. The chef outdid himself to make the required portions tasty and used different herbs and seasonings every day. Mr. W. discovered that he looked forward to and actually relished his daily cottage cheese salad, but didn't understand just why it was 'required eating.' It was not until his blood pressure registered normal without medication that the director took him aside and explained the effects and benefits of using linseed oil with protein-rich cottage cheese. Mr. W. has incorporated this simple meal into his daily diet and now finds his tolerance to stress has been immeasurably enhanced. He no longer has hypertension and his doctor has said he has conquered the risk of suffering a sudden heart attack or paralyzing stroke.

ATHEROSCLEROSIS—A middle-aged construction worker of 50, Mr. Hank C., was told by his doctor that his serum cholesterol was registering at a very high level and he was in danger of developing an arterial blockage which could result in a stroke or serious heart attack. This nutritionally-oriented and enlightened doctor outlined the dietary changes he wanted Mr. C. to make in his eating habits and emphasized the importance of including linseed oil and cottage cheese on the menu every day. Mr. C. carried the instructions home to his wife and she immediately visited the local market, made the necessary purchases, and began serving the exact meals that the doctor had prescribed.

After two months of healthy eating, including a daily salad of cottage cheese dressed with linseed oil, the doctor was very pleased to find that Mr. C's dangerously high serum cholesterol level had been significantly lowered and pronounced him free of the imminent possibility of a blockage-induced heart seizure or sudden stroke.

FAULTY METABOLISM—A young up-and-coming career woman of 33, Miss Georgine A., had been taking thyroid medication for many years on the advice of her physician, but still found herself grossly overtired, easily irritated, and continually fighting a tendency to put on weight. This attractive young women literally put herself on what was almost a starvation diet in an attempt to maintain a svelte figure. When she responded to what was a very real cry from her body for help and 'fell off her diet,' she gorged on saturated fats and sweets. When this happened, she often cried herself to sleep at night and fasted the following day in an attempt to make up for what she called her 'indulgence' the day before.

What Miss. A. viewed as a lack of willpower and indulgence was actually an attempt by her body to stimulate her into supplying the essential fatty acids and complex carbohydrates it required for healthy metabolism. Where she went wrong was in supplying heavily saturated fats and sugary carbohydrates instead.

One day as she was eating a hasty lunch of cottage cheese at her desk, she was joined by a co-worker who was having the same little meal. The co-worker took a vial of linseed oil from her handbag and proceeded to lace her dish of cottage cheese with it. Knowing this friend to be one who never 'dieted,' Miss A. questioned her about this 'strange practice' and was thus introduced to Dr. Budwig's ideas. We are pleased to be able to tell you that Miss A. now makes one daily meal of linseed oil and cottage cheese and says she 'never felt better' in her life. Her days of seesaw dieting are behind her; she has tremendous energy and is moving up quite steadily in her career.

A Simple Suggestion

It's hard to believe that simply supplying the body with a daily dose (one tablespoon) of raw, cold-processed, unrefined linseed oil with the good quality protein present in (one-half cup) cottage cheese can make such a vital difference in health, but the benefits of incorporating this simple meal into a diet are well documented and backed by sound research. The essential fatty acids (linoleic, linolenic) the body requires for healthy functioning and efficient metabolism of lipids (fats) are present in natural abundance in this ancient botanical, recently rediscovered.

As you have read in the foregoing material, scientists all over the world are quite rightly singing the praise of *Linum usitatissimum*: linseed oil. You just might want to consider the possible health benefits of adding a linseed oil dressed, herb flavored, enriched cottage cheese salad to your daily menu. Judging by the unprecedented results achieved in research, it must be said that dietary linseed oil has to be an extremely powerful natural preventive.

It always pains us to bring you important news of a medicinal or botanical that is not readily available in local stores. Correctly produced (raw, cold-processed, *unrefined*) linseed oil is difficult, if not nearly impossible, to obtain in the United States. The brand you want - *LINOSAN*™ - is imported and correctly produced to retain all its vital health-promoting properties. Major health food stores should have *Linosan,* but if you can't locate this crude linseed oil, please see the final chapter for the name of the U.S. distributor.

EDITORS NOTE—The material in this chapter is a prepublication release and has been excerpted from a new in-depth book on cancer entitled *How To Fight Cancer & Win* (Fischer Publishing Company, Canfield, Ohio 44406), still in manuscript form. The author believed that this information could be of such vital importance to the American public that it should be made available immediately and not held pending future publication. Note: *How To Fight Cancer & Win* carries additional material on linseed oil received too recently to include in this book.

CHAPTER 7

Migraine— Another Name For Pain

There Are Alternatives To Chemical Pain Relievers

THE MIGRAINE HEADACHE—Most medical authorities agree that migraines are the result of a central nervous system disorder which causes pressure in the arteries of the head. A migraine usually begins with a pain in the temples, eyes, or forehead which spreads to involve the entire cranial surface. As migraine sufferers know only too well, an attack may last several days or strike as a blinding pain of just a few minutes duration. When in the throes of a migraine attack, the victim may experience nausea, vomiting, constipation (or diarrhea), and is understandably irritable. Because the eyes are usually very sensitive to light, many migraine sufferers seek a dark room.

Directly before the pain begins, the arteries supplying the head with blood contract and blood flow is reduced. This constriction gives rise to either a flushed look (from the trapped blood) or a pallor of the face. The walls of the affected arteries swell, become tender, and may become temporarily rigid as excess blood accumulates. As the constriction diminishes, the throbbing pain intensifies with every heart beat. Typically, the eyes are swollen and red and may tear constantly. Dizziness and visual defects are common during an attack.

What Triggers A Migraine?

COMMON FOODS—Certain common foods are believed by many medical authorities to trigger a migraine attack. The food substances implicated include dairy products, chocolate, colas and other soft drinks, corn, onions and garlic, pork, eggs, citrus fruits, wheat, coffee, alcohol (especially the dark colored drinks such as red wine, rum, rye, scotch, and beer), cheese, chicken livers, pickled herring, canned figs, and the pods of broad beans.

At least one recognized health authority believes that an alkaline diet, with emphasis on all fruits except citrus, vegetables, and sprouts, is the answer. Giving credence to this theory is research coming out of Britain showing that some victims of migraine attacks are unable to process foods containing certain amines. These amines are present in excess in cheese, wine, citrus, chocolate and alcohol, already on the list of suspect foods.

FOOD ADDITIVES—If you are a lover of Chinese food and also suffer from migraines, you should know that *MSG* (monosodium glutamate) has been found to be the culprit in a number of cases. MSG is frequently used in oriental dishes, as well as being present in many commercially processed foods in U.S. supermarkets. Other additives that have been implicated in migraine attacks are the *nitrates* and *nitrites*. Cold cuts, hot dogs, bacon, and ham are usually processed with sodium nitrate or sodium nitrite. Check the ingredient panel to be sure.

It really isn't difficult to determine if a dietary factor is involved in migraine attacks. Keep a careful and detailed diary of every bite of food you eat during each 24-hour period for one week. A migraine can occur as long a 24 hours after eating the food that triggered it. If a migraine strikes, check your food diary to see if you have eaten any of the common food substances thought to trigger an attack. Eliminate any offending food from your next week's menus and continue keeping a diary until you are able to determine conclusively if a dietary factor is involved in your suffering.

HORMONES—The journal *Headache* (April 1975) reported on research conducted by Lee Kudrow, M.D. (Encino, California) on the relationship between hormones and migraines. Dr. Kudrow discovered that 70 percent of his female patients who had migraines had a measurable reduction of symptoms when they discontinued taking birth control pills. In a group of menopausal women taking estrogen supplements, close to 60 percent found their migraines diminished in intensity and severity when their hormone therapy was discontinued.

HYPOGLYCEMIA—Low blood sugar has been proven to trigger migraine attacks in many cases. (See *Sugar*, Chapter 4.) Ingesting a good diet of high quality protein and complex carbohydrates can completely eliminate migraines for borderline of full-fledged hypoglycemics. One trick that has been reported very successful in reducing the severity and number of migraines is taking a glass of milk (please select the low-fat variety) in the morning upon arising and in the evening before retiring.

CONSTIPATION—Chronic constipation is believed to play a large part in triggering a continuing series of migraine attacks. This all too common problem is easily corrected. Please see *Constipation* (Chapter 9).

LACK OF EXERCISE—Because the arteries supplying the head are involved in migraine attacks, many authorities believe the root of the problem is in the circulatory system. A regular exercise regimen which includes deep-breathing can be of immense help. Please see *Rebounding* (Chapter 1) for some fun exercise, and the *F-M Circulizer System* (Chapter 10) for a passive aid which stimulates circulation.

STRESS—It has long been noted that migraine headaches seem to afflict the individual who is tense and 'up-tight' more often than the 'happy-go-lucky' guy who refuses to let anything bother him. There are ways to cope with stress and nervous tension without resorting to prescribed tranquilizers. Please see *Conquering Depression & Handling Stress* (Chapter 19).

Relief Without Drugs

ACUPUNCTURE—The experts report real success in preventing the *occurrence* of migraine headaches with a series of acupuncture treatments. (Contrast this method with waiting for an attack to start *before* taking a pain killer.) *The American Journal of Chinese Medicine* showed that after 6 months of acupuncture, close to 70 percent of the migraine patients thus treated were able to discontinue their use of pain medication. Related symptoms (nausea, vomiting, the need to lie in a dark room, missing work because of pain) were reduced or completely eliminated in 82 percent. A two year study conducted at Northwestern University Medical School has verified the benefits of this ancient treatment.

Because blood flow has been shown to increase during a migraine attack, medical scientists theorize that acupuncture affects the blood circulation and acts to normalize it in some as yet unexplained way.

ACUPRESSURE—After the series of acupuncture treatments has been completed, patients are taught an acupressure technique that they can do at home as adjunctive therapy. The major acupressure point for migraine headaches is located on the lower part of the earlobe (the tail of the helix). At the onset of a migraine, place the thumb behind the lobe of the ear (on the involved side) and the index finger on the front of the lobe. Pinch the lobe between the thumb and index finger and rotate the index finger in a small circular motion. The severity of the attack determines how much pressure to exert.

AURICULOTHERAPY—Just inside the opening of the ear canal are two acupressure points that can be stimulated by medical practitioners knowledgeable in this art. This is *not* a home treatment. Using a small bent glass rod shaped rather like a little golf club, the doctor stimulates the special points, located along the bottom of the ear canal opening (the intertragic incisure). Although we don't have any statistics, good success in reducing the incidents of migraines and related symptoms have been reported.

SUPPLEMENTS—Many migraine sufferers can be helped by the addition of the following supplements to their daily regimen: Niacin, B-Complex, Pantothenic Acid, Magnesium, Brewer's Yeast, Rutin, Vitamin E, Selenium, and Vitamin C. Check with your doctor to determine your personal requirements. If you prefer a natural supplement please see *Bee Pollen* (Charpter 13). Bee pollen is a natural source of these important elements.

HAIR DRYER—Finding relief from a migraine with a hair dryer might seem far fetched, but it works for some. This method was reported at a meeting of the American Association for the Study of Headaches in 1974 by Dr. Charles Adler of Denver, Colorado. Dr. Adler says that if more of his patients continue to benefit, "someone will have to make up a complex theory to explain why." If you want to try this method, you need the type of hair dryer that has a bonnet. At the first suspicion of an attack, pop the bonnet on your head, turn on the heat, and relax.

HERBAL HELPERS—The medicinal herbs have been used since time immemorial for various conditions of ill health. To assist the nervous system and help overcome migraines, the following herbal teas are recommended by knowledgeable herbalists.

Herb Tea—Mix together: 1/4 ounce each Dandelion Root, Centaury, Wild Carrot, Ginger Root, Marshmallow Root, Motherwort, and Vervain. Simmer the blend in two pints of water for 15 minutes. Remove from heat and strain. Sip four ounces of the liquid before each of the three daily meals. You may add honey if you like.

The Headache Healer—Feverfew (Chrysanthemum parthenium) is *the* herb of choice for both serious mirgraine pain and the occasional headache that has you reaching for aspirin or some stronger over-the-counter pain reliever. Herbalists say the name is a corruption of *febrifuge*, medically defined as a substance which reduces fever and lessens pain. This plant is often found growing in fields, meadows, and hedgerows and attains a height of two feet or more. It bears small daisy like flowers of butter yellow with white rays around their outer perimeter. Feverfew's stems are of a downy texture with many short hairs, as are its leaves.

An old herbal says, "An infusion of the Feverfew flowers will allay any distressing sensitiveness to pain (even in an highly nervous subject) and will afford relief to the face-ache or earache of a dyspeptic or rheumatic person."

Europeans commonly employ Feverfew for headaches, nervousness, hysterical complaints, and depressions. An 18th century British herbalist tells of a young mother who had suffered all her life with "terrible and consistant headaches, fixed in one spot of the cranium, raging to distraction." The young aristocrat was completely cured when a house maid, fresh from a country farm, brewed Feverfew tea for her young mistress.

Using *Feverfew* as a base, the best herbal relief for migraine pain (and its root cause) is a combination of three of the medicinal botanicals. *Vervain* (Verbena officinalis) is noted for bringing speedy relief from all headache pain, mild or severe, whether it arises from congestion, tension, nerves, or the circulatory abnormalities of a rampaging migraine. *Rosemary* (Rosmarinus officinalis) is a valuable and pleasant addition to the blend. Master herbalist Parkinson said Rosemary elixir was a curative tonic "inwardly for the head and heart and outwardly for the sinews and joints."

To brew this natural migraine reliever at home, gently blend together 2 ounces each of Feverfew and Rosemary with 1 ounce of

Vervain. For each cup of tea, pour 6 ounces of freshly boiled water over one rounded tablespoon of the crushed dried herbs. Cover and allow the infusion to steep for 5 minutes. (Note: If you are using fresh herbs, finely mince (scissors make it easy) and use two rounded tablespoons for each 6 ounces of freshly boiled water.) Add honey to taste and sip hot. If a stuffy nose is adding to your misery, the juice of one-half lemon will aid in loosening the congestion.

Note: Unlike drugs, herbs work slowly to improve the internal workings of the body. The experts say that using this special blend over a period of weeks can result in a gradual lessening of the severity of migraine attacks, lengthen the period of the time between attacks, and reduce migraine related symptoms.

Tea & Sympathy

"Tea and sympathy are very nice but getting well is worth the price." Herbal teas and a sympathetic family may go a long way toward making a migraine attack a bit more bearable, but many victims of this condition believe nothing can ease the agony they must endure except strong prescribed pain killers. If you (or someone you care about) is subject to migraine attacks, please see if you can discover which of the known triggers has a loaded gun at your head. Investigate the migraine preventives we have compiled for you and try one or all of them. Be patient, however. Natural remedies work to normalize the body and correcting a long standing abnormality takes time.

If you are migraine sufferer, you have our sympathy along with the best treatments and preventives our research has been able to discover. And that's a lot more important than tea and sympathy in the long run.

CHAPTER 8

Varicose Veins

They're A Lot More Than Just Unsightly

Although more women than men develop varicose veins, this is not exclusively a women's problem. Varicose veins more often afflict the aging rather than young adults or middle-aged persons, but this is not exclusively a problem of seniors either. Support stockings may help ease the discomfort and certainly hide the ugliness nicely, but the condition may be a lot more serious than would appear at first glance.

As a matter of fact, complications arising from varicose veins can be extremely serious. Long-term varicosities may be accompanied by eczema and ulcers that can become large enough to affect the entire leg and which can eat clear down to the bone.

Varicose veins can develop into *phlebitis,* a swelling and inflammation of the veins with accompanying pain and tenderness along their entire length. This condition may give rise to a rapid pulse, pain in the joints, and a mild elevation in temperature.

If a clot (thrombus) develops in a vein, the condition can escalate into *thrombophlebitis,* a long way past the point where support stockings are useful. Your doctor will probably order bed rest and will want to cushion and elevate the affected leg. The danger, of course, is that the clot may break loose and cause a heart attack.

A CIRCULATORY PROBLEM—Varicose veins are directly attributable to impaired circulation. The venous valves in the veins of the legs work somewhat like the locks of a great canal used to transport huge vessels up to another level against the pull of gravity. In a lock, the water floating the ship is prevented from leaking out backwards while more is pumped in to raise the giant vessel to the next level.

The valves in the veins of the leg work against gravity to raise the blood level-by-level in order to return it to the heart and lungs for cleansing and oxygenating in much the same manner as the ship is raised. If the venous valves are crippled, the blood pools in the veins or even slips backwards a level or two. The veins stretch and expand under the pressure of the blood, making the upward return of the blood even more difficult.

With sluggish or impaired circulation, varicosities eventually occur and unsightly corded blue veins pop out and become visible near the surface of the skin. Unfortunately, that's only the tip of the iceberg.

The veins running near the surface of the leg carry only a small fraction of the venous blood. Around 80 to 90 percent of the veins which carry the blood to be returned are deep inside the legs muscles — and they are the ones first afflicted by impaired circulation. *When varicosities are visible near the surface of the skin, you can be certain that deeper veins are in even worse shape.* Nature expands the venous network and uses the superficial surface veins to carry the blood in order to ease the burden on the deep-seated veins you can't see.

Cause & Effect

LACK OF EXERCISE—A lack of exercise and indolent life style is the largest single factor contributing to the development of varicose veins. Regular exercise improves the entire circulatory system and stimulates the return of the venous blood, preventing it from pooling in the leg veins and creating pressure on the valves.

Specialists at the prestigious Mayo Clinic in Minnesota have been quoted as saying, "Exercise of the leg and calf muscles is essential for normal functioning of the musculovenous pumping against gravitational forces."

CONSTIPATION—Constipation and the straining that results create an abnormal amount of pressure which is transmitted to the leg veins. Studies show that this pressure causes a backup of the blood flow, leading to the initial failure of the valves. When constipation becomes a chronic condition and the colon is continually overfull and distended, more pressure is put on the veins running through the pelvis and into the legs. The straining which is necessary to pass a hard and compacted stool adds to the weakening of the valves.

CHAIR SITTING & POSTURE—How long we sit in one place has a lot to do with the development of varicosities. In the early 1970s, Dr. Colin James Alexander of New Zealand, publishing in the British Medical Journal, reported on the effects of allowing the edge of a chair to press against the blood vessels in the thighs year after year.

Although the leg veins sustain the greatest pressure when standing, most of us move around when we're upright and this movement actually helps circulation by stimulating muscular contractions. But sitting in a chair, even the most comfortable cushy one, results in constant pressure. According to Dr. Alexander, the pressure on the veins caused by sitting in a chair is more than twice that which is exerted when we're sitting on the floor.

As far as posture goes, crossing your legs in any fashion is a no-no. Perhaps your grandmother taught you that real ladies only cross their ankles, but certainly never put one leg over the other at the knee. Execpt among British royalty, failing to observe this little nicety from the last century is no longer considered the mark of a fallen woman. However, Mother Nature still frowns on this common posture fault and shows her displeasure with emerging varicosities. Crossing the legs adds considerably to the pressure on the venous system and impedes circulation.

PREGNANCY—Although rare in modern times, and we'll tell you why in a moment, pregnancy sometimes sets the stage for varicose veins. During childbirth, the pressure created by the babe's emerging head compresses the veins in the pelvis which carry the returning blood from the legs, *temporarily* incapacitating the venous valves. This effect doesn't last.

But not so very long ago, a woman was given bed rest following birth and told to avoid any undue exertion. Remembering that the veins depend on the muscles in the legs to push the blood upwards, it's easy to see why the longer the bed rest lasts, the more the returning blood stagnates and expands the lax veins. Nowadays, young mothers are encouraged to rise from their beds and walk. Varicose veins directly attributable to pregnancy are now very uncommon.

LIVER MALFUNCTION—The liver is the largest organ in the body and performs many vital functions. An abnormally enlarged, swollen, or fatty liver impedes the return of the blood to the heart and has been shown to be a contributing cause of varicosities. Improving the action of the liver with a cleansing program and good nutritional support has proved an effective adjunctive treatment for varicose veins.

LACK OF VITAMIN E—In the normal functioning of the body, Vitamin E works to dissolve and/or prevent the formation of blood clots. A long-term deficiency of this important vitamin has been tied to the development of varicosities. Some authorities believe that American women, in particular, are often seriously lacking in Vitamin E. Overprocessed and refined foods don't supply sufficient Vitamin E and many women routinely take an iron supplement. Iron can destroy Vitamin E stores in the body.

Prevention Beats Treatment

If ever a platitude fit the occasion, it's this one: "An ounce of prevention is worth a pound of cure." Varicose veins are ugly, painful, and a serious health problem. Following a healthy lifestyle and taking a few simple preventive steps *now* may mean that you can avoid this problem. Here's how:

EXERCISE—First, last, and always — the best way to prevent varicose veins is to exercise. If your job, your choice of relaxation, or your inclination keeps you sitting, you are risking developing varicose veins and all the problems that go along with them. Sitting too much or resting too much leads to sluggish circulation because the veins are largely dependent on the muscle contractions in the legs to force the blood upwards through the valves.

Because varicosities are residual pools of blood stagnating in the veins, any exercise that keeps the blood pulsing along through the circulatory system is all to the good. (See Chapter 1 for the superior health benefits of *Rebound Exercise*.)

If health reasons prevent your taking part in some of the more strenuous sports, a daily walk in the fresh air is within reach of all. If you like to sit and knit or rock and talk, try fitting a 30 minute walk into your daily schedule and see how much better you feel. Your legs will thank you and, if you coax a friend into joining you, you'll earn another thank you.

SITTING EXERCISES—If your occupation keeps you on the seat of your pants, a few simple exercises can help stimulate circulation and prevent varicosities from developing. The following exercises are recommended by the Georgetown University School of Medicine. Dr. Charles A. Hufnagel of that splendid university says these exercises will, "Prevent the pooling of the blood in the veins and accelerate the return of the blood out of the veins."

During long periods of unavoidable sitting, take an exercise break about every half hour, and

1) Bend your foot toward the leg 15 times each, flexing your ankles. You'll feel the pull in both your calf and thigh muscles.

2) Extend your legs straight out horizontally and then return feet to the floor. Repeat this procedure 15 times as rapidly as possible.

CHANGE YOUR DIET—Simply conquering chronic or intermittent constipation alone will go a long way toward making your life a lot more comfortable and will prevent undue pressure from developing into varicosities. Because a lack of fiber in the diet has been shown to be the major cause of constipation, adding additional fiber to your diet is the easy answer. (See *Constipation* (Chapter 9) for a remedy to conquer constipation forever.)

NUTRITIONAL SUPPLEMENTS—Although you will want to discuss taking any supplements with your doctor to make sure they're okay for your personal body chemistry, the following is a basic list of supplements that can assist in promoting a healthy body and preventing varicose veins:

1. *Bioflavonoids:* According to recent research, rutin and the other bioflavonoids are very useful in reducing the uncomfortable symptoms of varicosities. They act to strengthen the capillaries and promote elasticity. (See *Vitamin P,* Chapter 3.)

2. *Brewer's Yeast:* With its content of high-quality B complex vitamins, amino acids, and minerals (selenium and zinc), Brewer's Yeast provides important nutrients of great benefit. It may help those who are already the victims of varicose veins and aids in preventing their occurrence. Take up to 3 tablespoons of powdered yeast daily stirred into pineapple juice. (Pineapple supplies *bromelain*, an important enzyme that assists the immune system.)

3. *B-Complex:* A good quality high-potency Vitamin B Complex preparation will help stimulate the liver to optimum efficiency. Energizing the liver aids those who have varicosities and acts as a preventive as well.

4. *Vitamin C:* Besides fighting the common cold, this important vitamin strengthens the blood vessels and helps keep them elastic. Take up to 3000 mg daily.

5. *Dry-Brush Massage:* This little-known European health-promoting treatment can be very helpful in mild cases of varicose veins and, because it stimulates the circulatory system, can be a useful preventive as well. See *Dry-Brush Massage* (Chapter 14).

6. *Vitamin E:* Vitamin E is helpful because it acts to prevent and/or dissolve blood clots. It also increases the vital elasticity of the veins. Between 600 to 1200 I.U. (International Units) of Vitamin E may be added to your daily intake. Vitamin E (ointment or oil) can be gently massaged into the affected area. Vitamin E is very healing. (See Chapter 15.)

7. *Garlic:* Garlic helps keep clots from forming and asssists in dissolving those already in place. See *Garlic* (Chapter 5).

8. *Herbs:* Certain herbals contain properties which assist the circulatory system. Marjoram, Comfrey, Marigold, Yarrow, and Mistletoe are all recommended by herbalists as a specific for circulatory complaints, including varicose veins. Brew an infusion (tea) according to manufacturer's directions. A Comfrey poultice, applied directly to the affected area, soothes the pain and comforts a victim of varicosities.

9. *Lecithin:* Lecithin, the friendly fat fighter, helps prevent the buildup of cholesterol on arterial walls, thus improving the circulation of the blood. See *Nutrition for a Healthy Heart* (Chapter 18).

10. *Support Stockings:* Late in 1960, the Delaware Curative Workshop of Wilmington, Delaware mounted a study of the effectiveness of name-brand commercial support hose containing 10 to 24 percent elastic spandex fibers. This study determined that the pain of varicose veins was reduced and swelling went down considerably. Support hose strengthen the calf muscles and

assist the circulatory system as well.

11. *Surgery:* Surgery has to be considered the court of last resort and should only be used when all else fails. Why? Surgery does not correct the *root cause* of varicosities and, unless the cause is corrected and prevented from recurring, varicose veins can redevelop within a relatively short period of time.

12. *Wheat Germ:* Fresh wheat germ is an excellent natural source of all B vitamins and Vitamin E. Sprinkled on cereal, it's a nice way to supplement your diet with these important elements. Two to three tablespoons daily is the recommended amount.

13. *Zinc:* Just 50 mg daily has been shown to speed the healing of affected blood vessels. Regular use assists the entire circulatory system.

Summing It All Up

Varicose veins are not some mysterious affliction that descends on us by pure bad luck. Varicosities are the result of years of poor nutrition, leading to chronic constipation — plus a lack of regular exercise, leading to circulatory problems. Mother Nature does a wonderful job of trying to compensate for our bad habits by using the peripheral surface veins to carry the returning blood — leading to varicosities. All she asks is a little assistance. Making some simple changes in your lifestyle will prevent the development of varicose veins for a lifetime.

The Natural Food Alternative to
Constipation

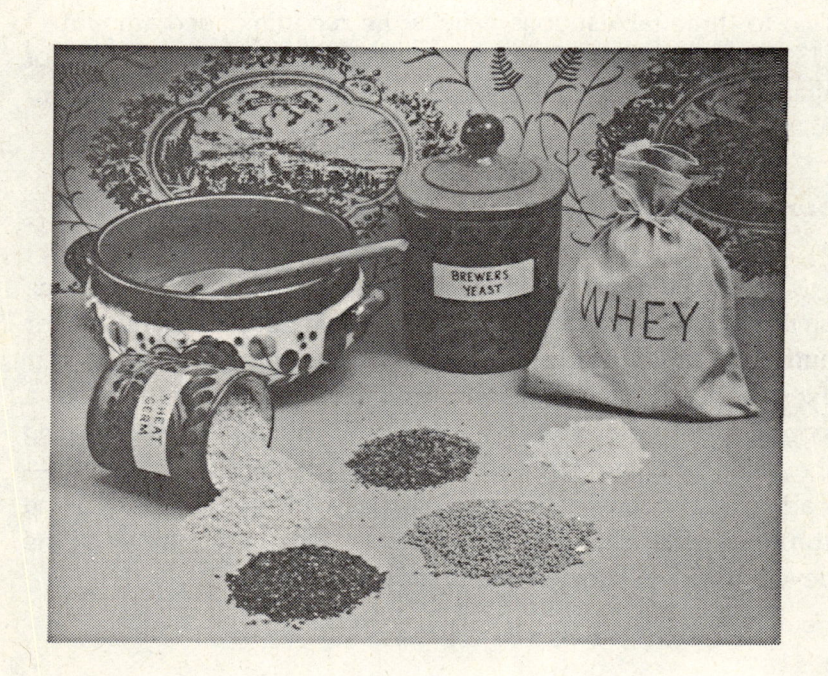

Chronic constipation is not only an often agonizing problem for many, but can also set the stage for other serious conditions of ill-health which may require medical treatment. This simple natural food and herbal kitchen recipe conquers constipation, establishes friendly intestinal flora, sweetens the bowel and encourages the peristalsis necessary for healthy normal functioning.

CHAPTER 9

Constipation

The All-Too Common Problem We'd Rather Not Talk About

IN FAVOR OF FIBER—Grandmother called it "roughage" and insisted you eat your cereal and fruit every morning, your sandwich at noon and your rice and vegetables every night. Back in grandmother's day, that might have been enough. The cereal and rice were unmilled, unrefined whole-grain, so was grandmother's home-baked bread and grandmother cooked vegetables with the skins on. "Saves vitamins," she said, "and besides, you need the roughage." Grandmother was right.

Today, medical authorities call it "fiber." In fact, your doctor may have said you need more fiber (cellulose) in your diet. But adding fiber to your diet isn't as easy as it was in grandmother's day. For instance, just 4 slices of whole-grain wheat bread will provide 30 grams of fiber, probably the optimum amount we need daily, but you would have to eat *16 slices of white bread* to ingest the same 30 grams of fiber. No wonder Grampa didn't need reading material in the outhouse! His digestive system and intestinal tract most likely functioned so efficiently he didn't spend much time there!

Now, you have to shop wisely to make sure the breakfast cereal and family bread you choose is made with the whole-grain. Make sure you select natural unpolished brown rice that still retains the fiber, rather than the snowy-white variety that invariably sticks to the pan from high starch content. Serve apples, peaches and pears unpeeled—the fiber's in the skin. Enjoy lots of high-fiber vegetables, such as beans, peas, broccoli and celery. And, for your health's sake, cook your potatoes in the jacket and eat the skins!

FIBER—WHO NEEDS IT?—We all do. Just about everyone will most likely benefit from extra fiber in their diet, In fact, research shows most of us need from four times to *ten times* as much fiber as we normally consume daily. The average daily intake of fiber from our processed, refined, denatured foods is around 4 grams. In so-called "uncivilized" countries, the daily intake averages about 30 grams, precisely the amount authorities recommend!

The intake of fiber markedly increases the growth of valuable organisms and the amount of B vitamins (particularly pantothenic acid), in the blood, urine and feces. Research shows the number of friendly intestinal bacteria is drastically decreased on a "smooth" diet lacking in fiber. Some individuals actually harbor intestinal bacteria which produce a B-complex destroying enzyme. This destructive bacteria is usually present in the stool of persons suffering from constipation.

Conditions of the digestive system and intestinal tract common to our western society include first and foremost, constipation, a national problem that continues to grow by astronomical proportions. Other disorders include appendicitis, diseases of the large intestine and rectum (including "irritable bowel syndrome"), hemorrhoids, cancer of the colon, diverticulosis and diverticulitis. Some authorities believe fiber may also affect the way in which your body processes fats and say fiber could be important in assisting to lower cholesterol levels in your blood stream. It is more than a coincidence that non-industrialized countries with a documented high-fiber intake have an enviably low incidence of these health problems.

FEAR OF FAT—As a nation, the United States is probably the most weight-conscious in the world. Literally, every third person age 16 or older is "on a diet" more or less permanently. Our books and plays, our magazines and publications, our television —and especially the advertising which continually bombards us— trumpets *"thin is in," "thin is beautiful," "thin is young,"* until we have been brainwashed into believing *only* thin is acceptable. In fact, *thin* has become a national paranoia.

In the public's collective mind, fiber equals carbohydrate, and carbohydrates equals "obesity." Nothing could be further from the truth, but it is entirely possible this erroneous thinking is the largest single contributing factor to the national problem of constipation.

FIBER IS "NO-CAL"—Your body does not digest fiber and it has no caloric or nutritional value at all. Fiber passes through the body virtually unchanged, but *supplies important bulk* needed by the intestines to carry away body wastes. This natural, bulk-producing ingredient of many foods stimulates natural intestinal movement. When your diet is deficient in fiber, your digestive process can become sluggish and you become constipated. *Fiber makes it possible for food to move through the digestive system and promotes normal intestinal function and bowel regularity.*

CONSTIPATION DEFINED—Constipation is correctly defined as the *abnormally delayed or infrequent passage of dry hardened feces*. It is important to understand that a bowel movement is *not* necessarily considered *"abnormally delayed"* if one doesn't occur naturally every day. Some persons may feel comfortable only if they evacuate their bowels daily, others may be perfectly comfortable doing so every other day and some every third day.

If the digestive system and intestinal tract are functioning correctly, the body maintains its own rhythm and doesn't require the stimulation of a laxative. It is only when the *discomfort* of an over-loaded bowel with rock-hard stool we must strain to pass occurs that we can rightly say we are constipated. Unfortunately, for too many of us, the embarrassment, discomfort and downright *pain* of constipation are a way of life.

CONSTIPATION—WHY IT OCCURS—Probably the most common digestive disorder is gas in the intestines. Efficient digestion and freedom from gas and attendant constipation depend on the production of hydrochloric acid, bile and digestive secretions and enzymes, on the type of intestinal bacteria present and the motility (movement) of the stomach and intestines.

For instance, when we eat too much, the secretions and enzymes of the digestive tract are overwhelmed and unable to efficiently process the excess amount of food we send down to the stomach. When the amount of food eaten at one meal is efficiently digested and absorbed, none remains to support the growth of undesirable bacteria and no gas is formed.

The broad purpose of the large intestines is to conserve water. The deficiency of certain vital nutrients that decreases the motility of the intestinal muscles may allow the intestine to reabsorb too much water, resulting in a dry, hard stool. The simplest way to avoid this type of constipation is to be certain your daily intake of food and liquid includes plenty of pure unadulterated water. Some authorities recommend as much as eight 8-ounce glasses of water be taken daily.

The importance of intestinal motility cannot be overemphasized. Rhythmic contractions of the muscles in the walls of the stomach and small intestines continue for hours after we eat—mixing the food mass with digestive juices, enzymes and bile acids—and bringing already digested food into contact with the absorbing surface of the intestinal walls. Without such contractions, foods will not be efficiently digested and absorbed.

If the involuntary muscle contractions of the stomach and intestine slow down or become intermittent, undigested food stagnates for hours (or even days) and so much gas forms that suffering may become acute. When the diet has been lacking in protein, Vitamin B1, pantothenic acid and the other B vitamins for a lengthy period of time, motility is seriously restricted and constipation—or worse—results.

A potassium deficiency, for instance, causes contractions of the intestinal muscles to slow down and, if the deficiency is severe, may even cause these muscles to become partially or completely paralyzed. This condition, which creates excruciating gas pains, is also associated with agonizing constipation. Fortunately, a potassium deficiency this severe is very rare and replacing the missing nutrients increases the motility of the intestines within a day or so.

Inadequate bile flow frequently causes constipation because undigested fats react with calcium and/or iron to form hard insoluble "soaps." Permanent correction of this type of constipation lies in increasing bile production. When your diet is low in protein and simultaneously high in refined carbohydrates, little bile is produced.

If the flow of bile is insufficient—or the gall bladder doesn't empty—or the liver isn't producing sufficient bile—fats remain in such large particles that enzymes cannot combine with them. Fat digestion is then incomplete and fat absorption is seriously reduced. When hard "soaps" form, the calcium and iron in your food fail to reach the blood and this causes constipation with overly firm, hard, dry stools.

Most fats from food melt at body temperature. But if bile is deficient, the melted undigested fats coat all foods and prevent the digestive enzymes from efficiently processing proteins and carbohydrates. Further, the lack of bile acids prevents the vital absorption of carotene and Vitamins A, D, E, and K. People with a sluggish gall bladder are commonly found to be deficient in linoleic acid, carotene and fat-soluble vitamins.

Intestinal bacteria multiply rapidly on undigested food, releasing quantities of histamines and gas, causing gas pains, constipation, halitosis and a foul-smelling stool. If your digestion is working efficiently, a healthy individual produces stool with little or no odor.

The constipation caused by inadequate bile flow is probably the most serious of all types. If this underlying condition goes untended, it can cause severe anemia, porous bones, spontaneous fractures and the crumbling or collapse of one or more vertebrae. Faulty elimination associated with gall bladder problems invariably indicates a major loss of vital minerals.

Spastic constipation, characterized by spasms in the large bowel, is documented to occur when deficiencies of calcium, magnesium, potassium and Vitamin B6 are combined with other nutrient deficiencies which result in faulty elimination. A lack of choline, essential to liver function and one of the B complex vitamins, has been shown to produce constipation. Other symptoms of choline deficiency, such as unexplained headaches, dizziness, ear noises and heart palpitations usually improve or disappear completely within ten days of adequate choline supplementation.

In the case of atonic (lack of physiological tone, especially of a contractile organ), colon, poor muscle tone interferes with the circulation of blood, slows normal lymph flow, inhibits digestion— and often causes constipation. Weak and inefficiently functioning muscles may even make it impossible to control urination or a bowel movement, resulting in an embarrassing accident. Weak muscles cannot properly support internal organs—and organs not adequately supported cannot perform their functions efficiently.

As muscles consist largely of layers of protein (with some essential fatty acids), these nutrients must be present in sufficient amounts to maintain muscle strength. However, the chemistry of the muscles themselves and the nerves which control them is so complex just about every nutrient known plays a part in their contraction, relaxation and repair.

When lack of muscle tone results in fatigue, gas distention and constipation (and perphaps even the inability to pass urine without a catheter), the taking of potassium chloride tablets (and Vitamin E supplementation) have proved effective. However, the average adult obtains ample potassium in his diet from fruits and vegetables, particulary cooked green leafy ones, and by avoiding refined foods.

An often-overlooked cause of chronic constipation is a psychoneurosis wherein the mind produces such anxiety the individual is unable to move the bowels. Well-nourished adults on excellent diets may sometimes suffer from digestive disturbances resulting in a serious and long-standing problem with constipation. When these individuals are closely questioned under the care of a psychiatrist, they are often discovered to feel lonely and unloved and, in most instances, had severe colic as a baby. The unconscious mind recreates the "colic" that brought love and attention to the child. Treatment may be with sedatives, tranquilizers or psychotherapy.

An obstruction is anything which interferes with the passage of the intestinal contents through the bowel. Fortunately, the most common cause is adhesions left over from a prior surgery. Symptoms are cramping and severe, sharp abdominal pain with distention and vomiting. If the obstruction has not completely closed the bowel off, this condition may respond to aspiration of the bowel contents with a long intestinal tube. If aspiration does not clear the obstruction promptly, surgery is necessary.

On the very extreme side, constipation may be a sign of obstruction of the colon caused by a tumor or cancer. Fortunately, malignant tumors are more rare than benign tumors, but both produce the same symptoms and both are treated by surgery. However, if constipation continues to the point where the individual is unable to pass anything and is in real pain, a complete physical examination and x-ray of the colon is very much in order.

A little-recognized side-effect of long term constipation may be the development of varicose veins and hemorrhoids. In fact, some researchers believe the major cause of varicose veins is actually faulty elimination. When an overloaded bowel presses against veins in the lower abdomen year after year, the valves in the veins gradually break down allowing a reverse flow of blood.

In peoples of the world eating a diet of unrefined, mostly raw foods, varicose veins and hemorrhoids (actually a form of varicose veins), are virtually unknown. Among the Zulus in Africa, for instance, only three persons in a population of 115,319 were found to have varicose veins while 10% of the entire population of Britain suffers from this unsightly and uncomfortable condition.

Scientists believe a return to the old ways of eating can help prevent, or even correct, the situation. A hundred years ago, the diet might conceivably have consisted of fruits, vegetables (mostly raw), meats, eggs, cheese, sour milks (acidopholous/yogurt), nuts and whole-grain breads and cereals with no refined or processed foods at all. This wholesome diet would surely prevent constipation as well.

Some lower abdominal pain may easily be confused with constipation. As a case in point, irritable colon, spastic colon and spastic colitis are medical terms and all refer to the same condition, which is functional and not organic. A common cause of lower abdominal pain is the irritable colon syndrome. Symptoms may include a cramping in the abdomen, bloating, the passing of gas and an uncomfortable distension of the area.

Once the diagnosis in confirmed, treatment of an irritable colon consists of reassuring the patient the condition is not serious, advising a bland diet and, occasionally, prescribing sedatives or tranquilizers. When intestinal gas or bloating is severe, relief is often obtained by use of a gas-relieving silicone derivative. Mucous colitis is merely a variation of the irritable colon syndrome with the same symptoms as outlined above, except a large amount of harmless mucus is passed with the bowel movement.

In its early stages, appendicitis mimics constipation. As the condition escalates, symptoms include nausea, vomiting and severe abdominal pain. The abdominal muscles become rigid and very tender to the touch, with any pressure causing much pain. Body temperature rises and the number of white cells in the body increases. An accurate diagnosis must be made by a physician on the basis of x-ray and white blood cell count.

RELATED CONDITIONS—Diverticulosis is a condition in which small pockets form on the colonic wall. Numerous small pockets may occur which give the appearance of grapes. These sacs form in a weakened area of the bowel wall, weakened somewhat as a balloon or inner-tube may have a thin area. Diverticulosis can be diagnosed only by an x-ray examination and is most common in persons who are constantly constipated and must strain to pass their stool. Unless a complication occurs, no treatment is necessary.

Diverticulitis is an inflammation or infection in one or more of the diverticulosis sacs. Symptoms are low, cramping abdominal pain, which may be mistaken in its early stages for constipation. If the condition progresses, chills and fever and even the development of a mass which produces an obstruction in the bowel can occur.

Again, diagnosis can only be made by x-ray. Treatment of acute diverticulitis consists of antibiotics and a liquid diet. Individuals who suffer from chronic diverticulitis must eat properly and work to develop good bowel habits. If symptoms persist or an obstruction occurs, surgery is indicated.

In the foregoing pages, we have only briefly examined the many causes of constipation. To go into a complete and medically technical run-down of the workings of the stomach, intestines and bowels, would take a book in itself. Suffice it to say that the digestive system, intestinal tract, colon and rectum collectively—and, for the most part, very efficiently—processes the food we eat, extracts the nutrients we need to function and then excretes the waste matter.

I am just now reminded of a delightful old gentleman I knew years ago. He had a pink and shiny bald head with a monk's fringe of white hair and an enormous old-fashioned handlebar moustache slightly yellowing at the ends. He was known in the neighborhood as "The Colonel," but his true name escapes me now.

I enjoyed chatting with him. The Colonel hadn't lost his sense of humor and his mind was as sharp as a tack. However, at 72 years of age, he suffered most dreadfully with chronic constipation and constantly groused his "digestive juices were all used up along with all the other juices that made life worth living." In the twilight of his life, he existed almost entirely on liquids and told me once, "At my age, a good bowel movement is better and more satisfying than sex ever was, at least as I remember it!"

If you are a sufferer of chronic constipation, you might echo that sentiment at times. Don't despair, dear reader, help is on the way! In the following sections we will explore the various types of laxative remedies and I will give you a kitchen recipe guaranteed to keep the pipes open and in good working order. Read on.

Lets Talk Laxatives
There Must be a Better Way

If you suffer from occasional constipation, you may be one of the many who ignore the condition in the hope it will go away. True, nature has a way of taking care of the problem and, if we just let nature take its course, relief may be just a day or so away. Or it may not.

On the other hand, the constipation may be so acute— and so painful—that the only answer seems to be to resort to a laxative that will relieve the problem. Judging by the sale of over-the-counter laxatives, this is the solution the majority of us favor.

More than 5,000 types of laxatives and cathartics are used in the United States alone. Americans spend more than a hundred million dollars per year on various treatments for constipation. Many of these laxatives contain harsh and even poisonous substances to cause the colon to react and eliminate them as rapidly as possible—and the fecal material along with them.

When the body is functioning properly, the food we consume passes through the stomach and small intestines in a relatively short period of time. The length of time required for passage through the large intestine is all-important. We want to hurry it along. When the movement of waste material slows down and becomes sluggish, harmful bacteria builds up and the mass can putrify. In many persons, the passage is too slow and constipation results.

Good bowel habits are essential to promote a clean digestive tract. Normal intestinal function demands we allow the bowels to move when they will. It may surprise you to know that the lower end of the intestine is of a size that requires emptying every six hours. However, through habit, most of us have trained our bodies to retain waste for 24-hours or more. When nature calls, the urge should be answered quickly to avoid developing the bad bowel habits which lead to constipation.

Constipation is so common that about half the adults in the United States suffer from this condition, either as a chronic complaint or as a once-in-awhile problem. Because it is so common most of us feel we know enough about it and usually treat ourselves with an overnight laxative—but the use of laxatives in itself can also create problems.

LAXATIVE DEFINED—The term *laxative* comes from the Latin and literally means "having a tendency to *loosen* or relax, specifically to relieve constipation." But far too many laxatives, instead of *loosening* or *relaxing* work on the "blast out" theory. They create an overpowering urge and the bowel expels its contents, usually hard and sizable, without regard for the relative lack of elasticity of the rectum. (Ouch!) Let's examine the various types of laxatives available.

MINERAL OIL—For more than 25 years, the American Medical Association has been preaching against the use of mineral oil, probably the most damaging of all laxatives in use. Yet some unenlightened physicians still prescribe it and many take it routinely for constipation because of its lubricating action. Consider these facts: Mineral oil decreases the body's ability to absorb calcium and phosphorus and mineral oil itself absorbs vitamins A, D, E, K and carotene from the nutrients in the intestines. In addition, mineral oil picks up the fat-soluble vitamins from liquids and tissues throughout the body. All these valuable vitamins are then excreted and lost.

STIMULANT LAXATIVES—Castor oil and laxatives containing *phenolphthalein* are considered stimulant (or contact) laxatives and work directly on the small intestines to promote a bowel movement. These purge-type laxatives are often used for complete bowel evacuation prior to x-ray or surgery and usually prior to an endoscopic examination of the colon as well. Occasional use under a doctor's care is necessary and not harmful, but regular home-use can cause an excessive loss of water and the body salts, resulting in a weakening of the body. Many popular over-the-counter laxatives are too harsh to be used regularly as self-treatment.

SALINE LAXATIVES—The old familiar standbys *milk of magnesia* and *epsom salts* are typical examples of saline type laxatives. This type laxative is attractive as it often produces rapid results just when we need it most. However, their action is too thorough and over-empties the bowels. What happens then? Because the bowel is empty, several days pass before a normal bowel movement is necessary. This sets the stage for a self-induced condition known as *rebound constipation.*

REBOUND CONSTIPATION—When occasional constipation occurs and one of the popular over-the-counter laxatives is taken, which usually completely evacuates the bowel, having a normal bowel movement the following day is an impossibility. The body may require as much as several days to extract nutrients and process waste matter before we once again feel an urge to move our bowels. It's important to understand this time-lag which commonly occurs after taking a laxative is *not* constipation, but just nature catching up after the body's normal routine is interrupted. Don't let *rebound constipation* fool you into taking another laxative the following day.

LAXATIVE ABUSE—Individuals who have the idea that it's not only necessary but *normal* to have a daily bowel movement are likely candidates for laxative abuse. This thinking can lead to over-frequent self-dosing with laxatives, which results in a lazy bowel. In time, bowel habits become abnormal and may even cease to function *without* the stimulation of a laxative.

THE DANGERS OF LAXATIVES—Abnormal bowel habits, described above, are not the only problems arising from the constant use of laxatives. Repeated misuse can lead to dehydration (excessive loss of water), loss of nutrients (proteins and vitamins), and loss of electrolytes (body salts), such as sodium, potassium and calcium. Further, laxative abuse has been shown to cause spastic colitis, gastrointestinal disturbances and even physical changes in the intestine leading to chronic diarrhea.

WHEN *NOT* TO TAKE A LAXATIVE—The occasional use of a laxative is not normally harmful, but there are certain times when laxatives *must not* be taken. If stomach cramps, nausea, vomiting or other symptoms of appendicitis are present, *do not* take any type laxative. If you do have appendicitis, stimulating bowel activity with a laxative could result in the rupture of an inflamed appendix.

INTESTINAL MANAGEMENT—Many authorities believe the most important thing we can do for our bodies is to adopt a health-building routine that promotes a clean intestinal tract. Some of the most important life-functions take place in the intestines. Waste material not regularly evacuated can be carried by the blood and lymph to every part of the body. There is a strong relationship between the cleanliness and health of the intestinal tract and the health of the body as a whole.

Establishing normal intestinal flora with normal bacterial activity is of primary importance to establishing normal bowel movements. The simple kitchen recipe for a natural food-laxative in the following pages is *the better way* for cleansing and revitalizing the bowel and conquering constipation forever!

The Better Way
The Natural-Food Antidote for Constipation

Babies do it. Birds do it. Animals do it and the natural-living so-called "uncivilized" people of the world do it. Anyone who has ever cared for a baby has to be aware of the sounds of satisfaction the little one gives forth as he fills his diaper after eating. The native disappears into the bush or jungle and returns relieved. The dog barks and scratches the door to go out after his dinner. Nature intended that we evacuate our bowels a short time after each meal. But—*most of us don't do it.*

Instead, for whatever reason, far too many of us put nature "on-hold" until a more convenient time. We may be away from home and dislike using a public facility. We may be in an important business meeting. We may be involved in a lengthy telephone call. We may be on the tennis court or playing softball at the company picnic. We may be stirring jelly or pudding on the stove that might burn. We may even be intensely interested in a television program and wait for a commercial before making a mad dash for the commode where we try to fit nature's call into a 2-minute station break.

Some authorities believe that over 90% of the "diseases of civilization" are fostered by improper functioning of the colon. In fact, many well-accredited sources believe a sluggish colon gives rise to conditions as widely diverse as appendicitis, tonsillitis, infections of the liver and gall-bladder, dysfunction of the heart and blood vessels, sinusitis, arthritis and even rheumatism. This century has seen an astounding increase in the number of surgeries and treatments for the various parts of the problems of the colon, including the rectum and the anus itself. Consider hemorrhoids, fistulas, the prostate and the killer—cancer.

Our modern way of life is a major contributing factor. Instead of a plain, natural diet, we now eat highly refined and demineralized foods, often on the run. We are subjected daily to the stress and strain of surviving on the "fast-track" in our highly "civilized" world. We're too "busy" getting on to take adequate exercise. And, possibly most important, we are otherwise occupied or we are too "polite" (or too self-conscious) to excuse ourselves when nature signals a need to evacuate our bowels and promptly take care of the situation.

When toxic waste material is left to stagnate in the lower bowel tract, the system becomes polluted and constipation (or worse) results. In time, a condition of peristaltic malfunction occurs in the bowel with the fecal matter becoming condensed and compressed and movements are infrequent and difficult. Peristalsis is "nature calling," the rhythmic waves of involuntary contraction of the intestines which forces waste matter through the passageway and out. Inconvenient or not, more and more medical researchers are saying we would be better off to emulate the natives and move our bowels as often as we eat a regular meal.

Incidentally, speaking of the natives and their healthy bowel habits for a moment, you might find it as fascinating as I do to know that certain tribes in Africa who eat with their fingers from a common pot have a stiff penalty for the individual who "forgets" and dips into the pot with his left hand—the hand is immediately chopped off! (This may be primitive, but it's a highly effective method of sanitation.) Why? *Only the right hand is for eating.* The left hand is for wiping the behind with a handful of leaves after the trip into the bush.)

Certainly all of the foregoing material has impressed on you the importance of a healthy intestinal tract. Fortunately, it's not impossible to correct a lifetime history of chronic constipation, a sluggish colon and abnormal bowel habits. In fact, the remedy we're going to lay out for you now will vanquish constipation forever and may even give you a new lease on life! I call it:

The Antidote To Constipation

This old recipe, which I have updated for ease of preparation with today's ingredients, was developed by my doctor-father, who preferred to treat his patients with natural herbs whenever possible. He used this traditional country remedy for many, many years in his practice with great success. Unlike chemical laxatives, this combination of natural ingredients can be used every day without the least harm or side-effects to the body. My family still takes it regularly and many of our friends have used it for years. It always works wonders!

I have named it the "antidote," because an antidote is something that relieves, prevents or counteracts the effects of poison. "Poison" is defined as something that through its chemical action kills, injures or impairs an organism, something destructive or harmful, an object of aversion or abhorrence, something that inhibits the activity of or course of a reaction or process. This *antidote* will relieve, prevent and counteract the effects of the *constipation* which may be *poisoning* our system. In short, this is the perfect description of this recipe and I'm delighted with it.

We want to avoid the need for the quick temporary relief provided by laxatives, enemas and colonics. We want to cleanse, feed and stimulate the intestinal tract to allow it to work normally and naturally on its own without outside interference. Using the proper natural foods, we will build up the body, clean it out and encourage the necessary peristaltic action to allow the bowels to work freely and properly. And that's just what The Antidote can do for you.

The first order of business in cleansing and revitalizing the bowel is to establish friendly intestinal flora. In any type of intestinal disorder, the intestinal bacteria needs normalizing. Without normal bacterial activity, we may suffer a gas attack, diarrhea, constipation or set ourselves up for the onset of serious disease. The healthy way to supply the body with friendly bacteria is by adding a *lactic-acid* product, such as whey or yogurt, to your daily diet.

WHEY—Whey, the watery part of milk left when the curds are removed, is rich in lactose, minerals and vitamins and contains lactalbumin and traces of fat. Whey is needed to feed the friendly bacteria in the intestines and colon, keeping it healthy and active, and to "sweeten" the bowel. It may be produced from either goats' or cows' milk and can be fresh or powdered. For our purposes, the Antidote contains powdered whey.

Fermented milks have been used as foods and beverages in many cultures for centuries. It is the action of *bacillus acidi lactiti* which causes milk to sour. When the bacilli convert the milk sugar into lactic acid, the growth of disease-producing bacteria ceases and the milk becomes more digestible in the bargain. Lactic acid is a strong neutralizer of putrefaction in the colon.

To demonstrate the neutralizing power of lactic acid, a researcher immersed a pound of tainted beef in a crock of buttermilk. After just a few days in the buttermilk, bacteriological examination showed no putrefactive bacteria present in the meat. Science has shown that disease-producing bacteria cannot thrive in an acid medium, proving the desirability of adding lactic-acid to the diet. *You will find whey powder is a prime ingredient of The Antidote.*

YEAST—Yeast contains almost no fat, starch or sugar, and its excellent protein sticks to your ribs, satisfies the appetite, and increases your basal metabolism. In fact, more nutrients are concentrated in yeast than in almost any other food. (Only bee pollen beats yeast in complete nutrient content. See Chapter 13.) Good nutrition is a necessity in overcoming constipation forever. Research has shown that a deficiency of certain nutrients can in itself be a cause of constipation.

The B vitamin *inositol* is a case in point. A hundred times *more* inositol than any other vitamin (except niacin) is found in the human body. Inositol is so important in the diet that when animals are put on a regimen lacking inositol, their hair falls out, they develop an eczema rash (dermatitis), abnormalities of the eyes (inositol is concentrated in the lens of the human eye)—and *severe constipation*. The good news is that all these conditions clear up when the diet is supplemented with inositol. Yeast is a particularly good source of inositol.

Yeast also is rich in *choline*, another B vitamin, which has many duties in the body. It is necessary for the synthesis of nucleic acid and for the production of DNA and RNA. A deficiency of choline has been shown to result in high blood pressure and accompanying strokes, hemorrhages of the eyes and nephritis (kidney disease). When individuals suffering from a lack of choline have been adequately supplied, headaches, dizziness, ear noises and *constipation* improved or disappeared within 5 to 10 days, with the blood pressure dropping to normal.

Although *niacin* is somewhat difficult to obtain in a normal diet, yeast is an excellent source. A person laboring under a niacin deficiency usually experiences persistent *constipation*. Simultaneously, anemia and digestive disturbances are apparent, as the stomach cannot produce sufficient enzymes, digestive juices and stomach acid for normal digestion. The intestinal tract is stressed and constipation can alternate with diarrhea. If the niacin deficiency continues, the individual exhibits personality changes and may become depressed and hostile.

A lack of *thiamin*, vitamin B1, causes digestive disturbances in a number of ways. Energy production is so faulty that contractions of the stomach can't produce the necessary hydrochloric acid for the normal digestive processes, proteins are incompletely digested, minerals stay insoluble and several vitamins are completely destroyed. Gas pain, flatulence and *constipation* are inevitable. If thiamin is not supplied quickly, more serious conditions result. Yeast supplies the thiamin the body requires.

Persons on a refined, denatured diet deficient in *potassium* quickly develop fatigue, listlessness, gas pains, *constipation*, insomnia and low blood sugar. Muscles become soft and flabby and the pulse becomes slow, weak and irregular. By far the greatest harm caused by a lack of potassium is the effect on the heart. Heart attacks are often associated with a low potassium intake. An excessive intake of sodium (salt) can produce a potassium deficiency even when it appears the diet is adequately supplied. Yeast is an incomparable source of needed potassium.

To sum it all up, yeast is a rich and concentrated source of complete protein, the B vitamins (inositol, choline and thiamin), niacin and the minerals (particularly potassium) necessary for peristalsis and clean intestinal functioning. *As you can see, yeast plays a very important part in the Antidote formula.*

WHEAT GERM—Although there are many varieties of wheat, the first true wheat plant came from the lands of Galilee in Israel. All the hundreds of varieties of wheat grown around the world are descended from this original grain, mentioned favorably many times in religious writings. The germ of wheat is a strengthening food for all animals, including man, and is a source of natural vitamins and minerals. The germ is particularly rich in Vitamins E and B and, like yeast, contains inositol, choline, niacin and thiamin. *Besides being good for you all over, wheat germ is specified in the Antidote formula to nurture the friendly acidophilous culture.*

PSYLLIUM SEEDS—In herbal lore, *psyllium* is considered a superior intestinal lubricant and aid to the digestive tract. As a hydrophilic mucilloid, psyllium is often recommended by physicians because it is gentle, effective and virtually without the harmful side effects of chemical laxatives. Psyllium provides bulk (Grandmother's "roughage") with natural dietary fiber and absorbs large quantities of water to form a gel which softens the stool. Psyllium is considered to be an excellent colon and intestinal cleanser and healer, strengthening and toning the tissues. It does not irritate the mucous membranes and the intestinal tract is nicely lubricated for a smooth passage. *With these outstanding qualities, you might expect to find psyllium in the Antidote. It is.*

FLAXSEED—Flaxseed is another favorite of the master herbalists of the last century. It is a soothing natural laxative and provides additional fiber. Flaxseed can stimulate peristalsis and the glandular secretions necessary to normal intestinal functioning. This herb is so gentle, it has been given to sickly babies for its blood enriching properties. It is said to heal the body as it nourishes and is soothing to the throat, the linings of the intestines and the entire digestive tract. *Flaxseed is included in the Antidote for its healing qualities and gentle laxative action.*

In addition, these two important herbs are said to aid in cleansing waste matter from the liver, gall ducts and alimentary canal. Both psyllium and flaxseed encourage necessary bile secretions into the duodenum and help normalize the peristaltic action of the bowels.

MUSTARD SEED—Animals in the wild instinctively seek out and eat the mustard plant, presumably recognizing it for the fine tonic, disinfectant and digestive aid it is. Mustard seeds promote a healthy appetite, stimulate salivation (saliva acts upon food as we chew and is the first part of the digestive process) and the secretion of vital digestive juices. *Mustard seed helps eliminate intestinal gas and , with its other properties, this powerful little herb is an* *excellent optional addition to the Antidote.*

Experiments with animals have proved an unbalanced diet shortens the lifespan in one way or another. Indications continue to accumulate showing that an improper diet may actually shorten the life expectancy of man as well. Establishing a pattern of constipation and the resultant over-use of laxatives which leads to abnormal functioning of the intestinal tract is just one way we abuse our bodies. The food we eat, its type, its elements and the amounts in which we take it, have a profound effect on our body, our intestinal tract, our degree of health and well-being and our general fitness.

The natural way of conquering constipation forever is the major objective of The Natural-Food Antidote for Constipation—and that's just what it will do for you. I have attempted to analyze this recipe as completely as possible and my analysis shows that the specific nutrients required to cleanse and sweeten the bowel, encourage peristalsis and establish (or re-establish) good bowel habits are present in the formula.

Bon appetit!

The Natural Food Antidote For Constipation

1 cup Whey Powder
1½ cups Brewer's Yeast
1 cup Wheat Germ
½ cup Psyllium Seeds
½ cup Flaxseed
½ cup Mustard Seed*
(*Mustard Seed may be eliminated if not readily available)

All of these ingredients can be easily purchased at your local health-food store—or try a country co-op for lower prices. Both wheat germ and Brewer's yeast can be used in flake or powder form, but do purchase the whole seeds. Psyllium seeds, flaxseed and mustard seed should not be *powdered*, but *used whole*.

Simply mix thoroughly with your spoon in a big bowl until the blend is uniform. We suggest you mix up a two to four weeks supply (1 to 2 pounds). The mixture stores well in a plastic bag (with a twist tie) or jar, but always keep the lid tight. (The above recipe will produce approximately a 2 week supply for two people.)

Place 1 or 2 tablespoons of the mixture in a cup with the beverage of your choice (tea, milk, coffee or water) and swallow slowly. Additional liquid is advisable. Always rinse *the Antidote* down with a second glass of your favorite drink. Or just put a spoonful in your mouth and wash it down with plenty of liquid.

We suggest you take one or two tablespoons before meals, depending on your condition. You be the judge. Allow one or two days for results. Remember, this is *not* an overnight chemical blast, but a gentle food laxative that will correct faulty bowel habits and conquer constipation forever. In the beginning, it may take two or three days before a normal healthy bowel movement is evident. This Natural Food Laxative is also a very fine health breakfast. It is low in calories, easy on your stomach and helps prevent indigestion, as well as encouraging peristalsis of the intestines and promoting bowel regularity. This mixture of special stool-softening herbal ingredients activates the intestines and supports the natural, normal functioning of the bowel.

Tip: Authorities agree eating foods raw or lightly cooked, using whole grain breads and cereals rather than bleached white flour products, taking complex carbohydrates with natural sugars (fruits rather than pastries), and drinking plenty of water daily to flush out impurities will go along way toward fixing whatever ails us—including constipation!

CHAPTER 10

The F-M Circulizer System

New to the U.S - European Herbal Therapy

THE HERBAL FOOTBATH—After reading this chapter, you'll become aware of how advanced the overseas medical community is in the use of herbs. We have been searching the world investigating alternative forms of health therapies to bring back to the U.S. In our travels, we discovered a very important herbal treatment that is virtually unknown in America. For over 40 years, health specialists abroad have been using selected herbal essence blends with a temperature-controlled footbath device to *influence the vital blood circulation system* of the body. This chapter will be the first introduction of the temperature-controlled herbal footbath system for the American public.

The F-M System

THE UNIT ITSELF—This treatment system consists of a self-contained unit which the user fills with water and a prescribed herbal blend. But the real secret of this incredible device is the precise gradations of temperature that are preprogrammed into it. This clever machine first heats the water to the necessary temperature. Then the device gently raises the temperature of the water very gradually until the full power of the botanical essence has been released, thus insuring absorption of all medicinal properties.

Science has determined that the benefits of the prescribed herbs, when combined with this graduated and precisely controlled rise in temperature, are immeasurably enhanced. Tests have shown that the combination of herbs and the gradual rise in temperature greatly influences the entire circulatory system, the vascular system, and the inner organs of the body as well.

HERE'S HOW IT WORKS—The explanation is simple. In scientific circles, this phenomenon is know as the *'Dastre-Moratsche'* or *'consensual'* reaction. A good example of this reaction is the person who goes walking on a cold winter day. Let us suppose he inadvertently breaks through a thin film of ice covering a stream of almost frozen water which is deep enough to thoroughly soak his boots and the socks beneath. Because he has drastically lowered the temperature of the sensitive thermal receptors on the soles of his feet, he very soon develops a serious head cold. Even though his feet are far removed from the mucous membranes of his nose and sinus cavities, they are affected by this change in temperature. Measurements show that the temperature of the mucous membranes of the velum, oral cavity, and outer auditory canals drops when the feet are cold.

On the other hand, the temperature-controlled herbal footbath with its slowly rising temperature results in a beneficial effect that works by first expanding the tiny capillaries in the soles of the feet. As the temperature rises, the deep-seated larger arterioles and then the big blood vessels of the feet expand. Very soon, all the blood vessels of the feet are expanded to the maximum and this expansion effects travels upwards throughout the entire body, including the head region, carrying with it the medicinal properties of the herbs as they are absorbed.

Circulatory Complications Are Many

CONDITIONS BENEFITED—Some of the conditions successfully treated with herbs and the controlled temperature device include: influenza, colds, bronchitis, angina, bladder infections, asthma, migraine headaches, circulation problems, intermittent claudication, high cholesterol and triglyceride levels, rheumatism, dizziness, insomnia, eczema, psoriasis, arthritis, kidney problems, atherosclerosis, arteriosclerosis, osteoporosis, both high and low blood pressure, senility, varicose veins, glaucoma, hypercalcemia, angina pectoris, heart arrhythmia, impotence, lupus erythematosis, gangrene, prostrate problems, and on and on.

Extensive medically-supervised tests show this system to be a revolutionary approach to many health problems related to or complicated by poor circulation. In modern society, poor circulation is a universal problem, even in younger people. Many illnesses are associated with circulatory impairment. Circulatory problems are especially evident with advancing age. This herbal footbath can be used by anyone of any age in the privacy of the home. As an aid to stimulating circulation, it promises to be an effective preventive and prophylactic treatment to assist in overcoming existing illnesses and/or to guard against circulatory complaints.

Empirical Evidence Abounds

THE TESTIMONIALS POUR IN—If this method of treatment seems too good to be true, read on. From the files of various physicians comes a wealth of empirical evidence. The results detailed in the following stories of grateful patients will convince you.

Consider the case of Mrs. Marie B., an 84-year old woman suffering from arthrosis deformans of hip and knee joints. Her condition was subsequently complicated by gall stones, cystitis, and peritonitis. After an emergency operation (at age 82) which resulted in the removal of 8 feet of bowel, Mrs. B. was bedridden. After many months, she was eventually able to drag herself around painfully with the aid of crutches. Thrombosis and an embolism of the lung followed, but still she survived in spite of the fact that her doctors considered her case hopeless.

A series of treatments with the herbal footbath restored this woman almost miraculously. Mrs. B. herself says, "My health is better now than it was 20 years ago and I feel much younger! To me, these herb footbaths are a real Fountain of Youth. All my illnesses have gone. My friends often ask, "What is it that keeps you young?" I tell them that my blood is circulating again the way it did when I was in my teens and all the impurities that were making me sick have been flushed out of my body by the prescribed herbal blend. This method works excellently and is well worth the cost!"

The treatment of an 83-year old male patient suffering from hypertrophic prostatitis, George H., was complicated by a dangerous heart condition that precluded surgery. To further add to Mr. H.'s problem was the fact that the gland had enlarged to the size of a hen's egg. Because even the most weakened heart is not endangered by the therapeutic herbal footbath, this gentlemen was started on the baths immediately. After a four-week course of therapy, the enlargement was found to have vanished completely. Mr. H.'s medical doctor confessed to being amazed, so sure was he that the condition would only grow worse.

A 57-year old man who also suffered from an enlarged prostate had borne the condition for ten years before he was introduced to the herbal footbath. Thomas C.'s condition had progressed to the point where he was unable to urinate for some days and his doctor was considering the use of a catheter to afford him relief. Incredibly, just one herbal footbath dissolved the blockage within fifteen minutes. Mr. C. is continuing with therapy to insure that his prostate remains normal.

A registered nurse by the name of Rebecca W. was the victim of terrible headaches caused by a serious frontal sinusitis condition which had plagued her for over ten years. She spoke of feeling as if her eyes were being pulled from their sockets and was terrified because she felt she was going blind. Miss W. says, "These headaches were so violently painful that at times I actually considered suicide to escape the agony."

As a trained nurse, Miss W. was skeptical of the herbal footbath, but agreed to try a series of treatments in what she frankly called "pure desperation." The first few baths brought her no relief, and she had to be persuaded to continue. But after the sixth bath, her infection broke and she began discharging thick globs of pus from both nostrils. This foul-smelling discharge of pus continued for about ten days. After her thirteenth footbath, the discharge disappeared along with her violent headaches. Miss W. says, "I'm a true believer now. In fact, I advised a friend who also suffered from a severe sinus condition to take the baths and she, too, has been completely cured. We are both so thankful. Many people don't understand the agony a chronic sinus infection can cause. It's hard to describe the joy I feel about what this simple therapy has accomplished!"

For over twenty-nine years, a professional man in his mid-fifties had suffered from severe asthma and a serious cardiac weakness. Paul Y. was medically treated with injections for both asthma and his heart. He regularly inhaled a bronchodialator compound in order to breathe comfortably. Mr. Y.'s condition went from bad to worse. He was being transported via ambulance to a full-care facility when he lapsed into unconsciousness. His heart stopped beating and he was turning blue when a strong injection directly into his heart roused him just in time.

Fortunately, a health care specialist trained in the use of the herbal footbath took an interest in his case. Mr. Y. was treated therapeutically with prescribed herbs and the controlled-temperature footbath. After fifteen treatments, his asthma disappeared and his heart complaint was eased to the point where Mr. Y. is once again working at his profession. He now takes precautionary maintenance treatments.

A man of 43 years, Mr. Ludwig F., developed a serious case of scabies and was advised by his doctor to use a prescribed liquid for relief. Mr. F. found that the condition worsened instead of getting better. He was to the point where the only relief he found from the intolerable itching and pain was to scald himself in the shower.

After consulting a naturopathic doctor, Mr. F. used medicinal herbs and the footbath system. Just three days later, the itching began to ease and within a few days, Mr. F. was completely cured.

The herbal footbath was recommended to Mr. John B., 74 years of age, for a kidney condition. As a cigarette smoker for some sixty years of his life, Mr. B.'s circulation was understandably impaired. Although he had been told by many doctors over the years to stop smoking because it was seriously undermining his health, Mr. B. did not do so. At this writing, he has had only two sessions on the bath and it is too early to judge results as they apply to his kidney problem.

However, after just these two herbal bath treatments, Mr. B. reported in amazement that he had lost all desire to smoke and refused a cigarette when it was offered to him! (Note: This system has not been tested as a deterrent to smoking. Without further evidence, we must consider Mr. B.'s testimony as a purely personal statement which applies in his case alone, but we can conjecture that his system was purged of addicting nicotine. His case presents an interesting premise that should be explored further.)

Other grateful patients have written of their experiences using the herbal footbath as well. We include here excerpts from a few letters:

"We are convinced of the good effect of the herbal footbath. My husband is completely cured of the rheumatism that made him miserable for 20 years." N.M

"I had been suffering with varicose veins for many years and the pain handicapped me greatly. After twenty herbal footbaths, I was completely cured and all complaints connected with my varicose veins are gone. I stand eight hours a day at work, but the varicosities have not returned. I recommend the baths to everyone." B.L.

"As a nineteen-year old girl, I was made very unhappy because my face was disfigured with terrible acne. My doctor told me to eat a lot of fruit, cut down on the fat in my diet, and prescribed some herbs to use with the footbath. I did just what he told me to do." (Note: This young woman had the worse case of acne I have ever seen with eruptions the size of a nickle covering her face and back.) "I was so afraid I'd be scarred for life, but even the deep pits seem to be clearing. After two months, my skin is clear and soft and has a healthy look. I can't tell you what a difference this has made in my life!" S.D.S.

To Stimulate Circulation & Flush Away Toxins

THE PRESCRIBED HERBAL BLENDS—When used with precisely prescribed medicinal herbs, the controlled-temperature footbath system both improves vital blood circulation and works to flush the toxins out of the body. It is a medical fact that the skin is the largest eliminative organ of the body. Many impurities are excreted through the pores of the skin, carried outside along with the perspiration that helps regulate the temperature of the body. To understand this process, consider the stale smell of an unwashed body. Your nose tells you of the impurities collected on the surface of the skin which need to be washed away.

This premise is confirmed by the use of the herbal footbath. Very often patients undergoing treatment will complain of a sick stench coming from their skin. They should rejoice! This odor is proof-positive that the impurities and toxins contributing to a condition of ill health are being gradually eliminated. The skin is doing its job superlatively!

Another virtue which must be exercised in the use of the controlled-temperature herbal footbath is that of patience. It is unreasonable to expect immediate results from this natural form of therapy. If you have lived in this polluted and imperfect world for 20, 30, or 50 years, your body has unavoidably been accumulating toxins for 20, 30, or 50 years. When the impurities get stirred up and the healthy red blood begins coursing through your veins again as it did when you were a child, improvement is steady and sure.

For more information on how to order this unit, contact New Dimensions Distributors listed at the back of this book.

The Prostate

What It Is & What It Does

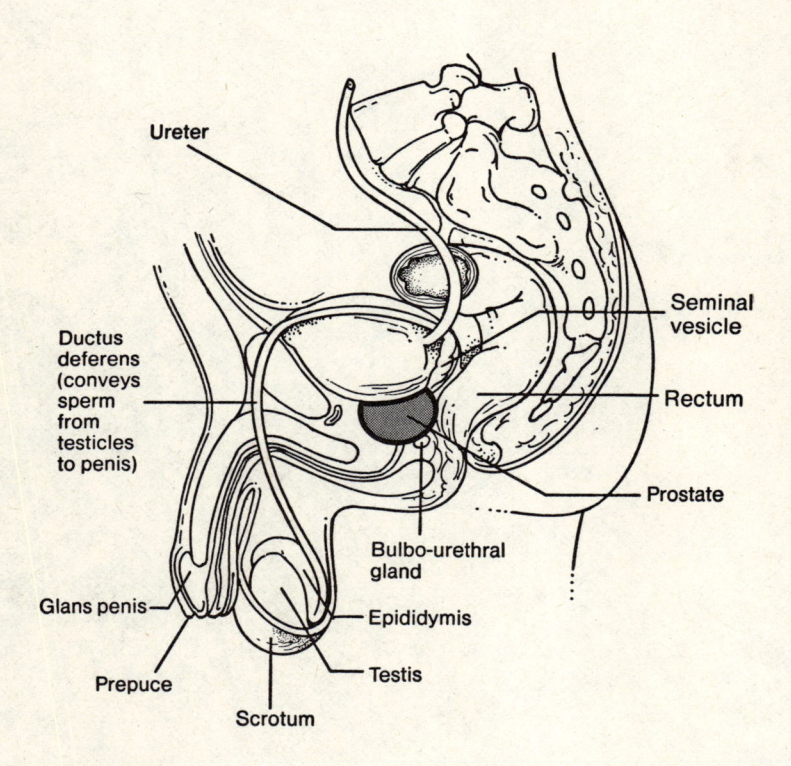

The male reproductive system is an incredibly complex piece of engineering — and just about everything that makes a man *male* is controlled by the prostate gland. Every man needs to know how to support the functioning of this very important gland, and what to do when things go wrong.

CHAPTER 11

Understanding The Prostate

Everything You Need To Know About This Vital Male Organ

THE GLAND ITSELF—The prostate is an organ approximately 1-½ inches in size located directly beneath the bladder in the male. This mighty mite weighs only around one ounce, but is vital to a healthy normally functioning male. The prostate has three ducts which open into the *urethra*. The urethra is the canal through which both urine and seminal fluid travel to exit from the penis. It is the prostate which stores the sperm and produces seminal fluid. This important gland contributes from 15 to 30 percent of the seminal fluid (semen) the male discharges during orgasm and it controls the muscles that cause ejaculation. In addition, the prostate controls the muscles used in passing urine. It is because the gland partially surrounds the urethra that any abnormal enlargement of the prostate affects normal urination and ejaculation.

The prostate gland is dependent on the male hormone *androgen*, which is secreted by the testicles (*testes*), for growth and development. (Incidentally, males who do not secrete an adequate amount of androgen may require injections of this male hormone to maintain normal functioning.) It is the testes which produce the spermatozoa needed to fertilize the female egg. The testes pass the sperm on to the prostate, which adds some necessary ingredients of its own, including a waxy substance which protects the sperm against the high acid content of the vagina. Without this protective covering, the acidity of the vagina would be fatal to the sperm.

The prostate produces seminal fluid constantly at a rate of about 5 to 30 drops every hour. During sexual excitation, production is increased. The liquid produced by the prostate contains the food supply needed by the sperm (150 million to 400 million) and also makes it possible for sperm to swim up the vaginal passageway. If an excess of seminal fluid is produced, but not ejaculated, it is voided a little at a time during urination.

During full sexual arousal leading to orgasm, the prostate initiates a rhythmic series of contractions around the urethra which triggers ejaculation as the male reaches his climax. Three or four bursts of semen are expelled at intervals of about one second apart. The muscles of the prostate alternately pump and contract with great force in order to propel the sperm-laden fluid deep into the vagina.

The prostate reaches mature size at puberty, but at around the age of 50, both the size of the prostate and the quantity of the secretion decreases. As a normal male ages, changes occur gradually in the prostate. Between the ages of 40 and 60, the gland slowly atrophies and fibrous tissue replaces the normal tissue. By the time a male passes his 60th year, the entire organ has been largley replaced by fibrous tissue.

Examining Prostate Disorders

AN OVERVIEW—In the male's later years, enlargement of the prostate is very common. An enlarged prostate often causes a compression of the urethra with subsequent difficulty in urinating. Inability to empty the bladder may cause the retained urine to stagnate and become infected. Uremic poisoning then becomes a very real danger.

Chronic prostate disorders are increasing yearly in the U.S. But by far the greatest hazard the male may face is cancer of the prostate, on the rise and one of the more common forms of malignancy. Upwards of 20,000 American males die of prostate cancer every year. Except for lung cancer, prostatic cancer afflicts males more than any other form of malignancy. Approximately 60,000 new cases are diagnosed in this country every year.

Unfortunately, statistics show that the average male will experience some type of prostate problem by the time he reaches age 50. After that age, one out of three will have a serious prostate problem that requires medical attention and at least one out of twelve will develop cancer.

CHRONIC PROSTATITIS—The diagnosis of chronic prostatis is difficult because the patient seldom runs a fever and very often no bacterial cause can be discerned. Symptoms include a need to urinate frequently and many sufferers of chronic prostatis lose their desire for sex. At times, the man may be impotent and unable to sustain an erection.

ACUTE PROSTATITIS—This condition stems from a bacterial infection of the prostate gland and is common in both young and older men. The male will have pain at the base of the penis and urination may be painful as well. The male typically feels his bladder has not been completely emptied even after urinating. Drops of a cloudy fluid may collect at the end of the penis, a problem also associated with certain venereal diseases. The male afflicted with acute prostatitis usually develops a high fever quite suddenly alternating with chills.

PROSTATIC HYPERTROPHY—*Benign prostatic hypertrophy* is an abnormal enlargement of the prostate gland entirely unrelated to cancer. The onset of symptoms occurs gradually over a period of years and is almost unnoticeable in the early stages of this condition. As enlargement progresses, however, the male will experience pain in the region of the prostate gland and may complain of lower back pain and discomfort when sitting. As the condition escalates, urination becomes a painful necessary function. The patient typically describes the pain as a burning sensation.

With further enlargement, the stream of urine that exited so forcefully during his early years now becomes a feeble trickle. The bladder continually feels uncomfortably full, which it is, and the victim must get up several times a night to drain off whatever he can in order to obtain a little relief.

When the male is able and engages in intercourse with an enlarged prostate, he usually experiences pain during ejaculation. He may suffer intermittent periods of impotence or, even though his control during sexual arousal in his younger years was excellent, he may ejaculate prematurely. Let's examine why an enlarged prostate causes all these very disturbing symptoms. Remembering that the urethra is partially surrounded by the prostate, it's easy to see that an abnormal enlargement of the gland acts to compress the urinary canal, thereby reducing the stream of urine to a dribble. The problem is further complicated because the enlarged prostate, with nowhere else to expand, pushes upwards against the bladder itself and narrows the duct which routes the urine into the urethra.

In its exterme manifestation, this condition can become life-threatening. You should certainly not allow prostatic hypertrophy to reach this stage without medical intervention. Here's what can happen. If the abnormal growth of the prostate continues unthwarted, the enlarged gland can completely close off the flow of urine through normal channels. The contents of the overfull and distended bladder may then become infected and/or back up into the kidneys, giving rise to a condition call *hydronephrous* which can seriously damage the function of the kidneys themselves. It can also lead to a severe inflammation of the bladder, *nephritis* (kidney inflammation), and *uremia* (uremic poisoning). This is a serious toxic condition caused when the kidneys can no longer excrete toxins and it can progress to complete kidney failure.

PROSTATIC CANCER—Cancer of the prostate is one of the most common forms of all malignancies. The affected area is usually hard and dry with small hidden islands of yellow cancer cells dotting the tissue. The cancer may show symptoms pointing the physician directly to the prostate, or it may cause no symptoms in the gland itself but metastasize (spread) to other parts of the body.

The malignancy can invade the bladder and the reproductive ducts leading into the prostate. Typically, the spinal and pelvic lymph nodes are first attacked, but cancer colonies may later develop in the chest and shoulders, liver, lungs, and/or bone by way of the blood circulatory system. About 70 percent of all prostatic cancer patients have bone involvement, usually discovered during autopsy. Prostatic cancers commonly develop on the area of the gland near the rectum and can often be identified early and quite readily by a rectal examination. Because this type of cancer seldom produces physical discomfort until it is well advanced, a regular yearly rectal examination is a must for males over the age of forty. During a rectal exam, your doctor will introduce a *sigmoidoscope* into the anus. This is a lighted instrument about 10 inches long which allows him to view the entire rectal area. Don't let your fear or embarrassment keep you from submitting to a rectal exam. It takes only 10 minutes, is virtually painless, and could save your life.

If your doctor discovers a hard nodule in the prostate gland, he will take a small snip of the suspect tissue for analysis. You should know that about half of the growths thus analyzed are cancerous. Early diagnosis is extremely important if treatment is to be successful. Most medical authorities agree that surgical removal of the prostate gland is indicated in the presence of cancer. It is important that you thoroughly understand any procedure your doctor recommends. Insist on a full and frank discussion of all options open to you.

THE TOTAL PROSTATECTOMY—After the complete surgical removal of the prostate gland, certain side effects are unavoidable. Because the prostate controlled the muscles used for urination, urine leakage should be expected for a few days until other controls take over. This effect will disappear along with any irritation in the area.

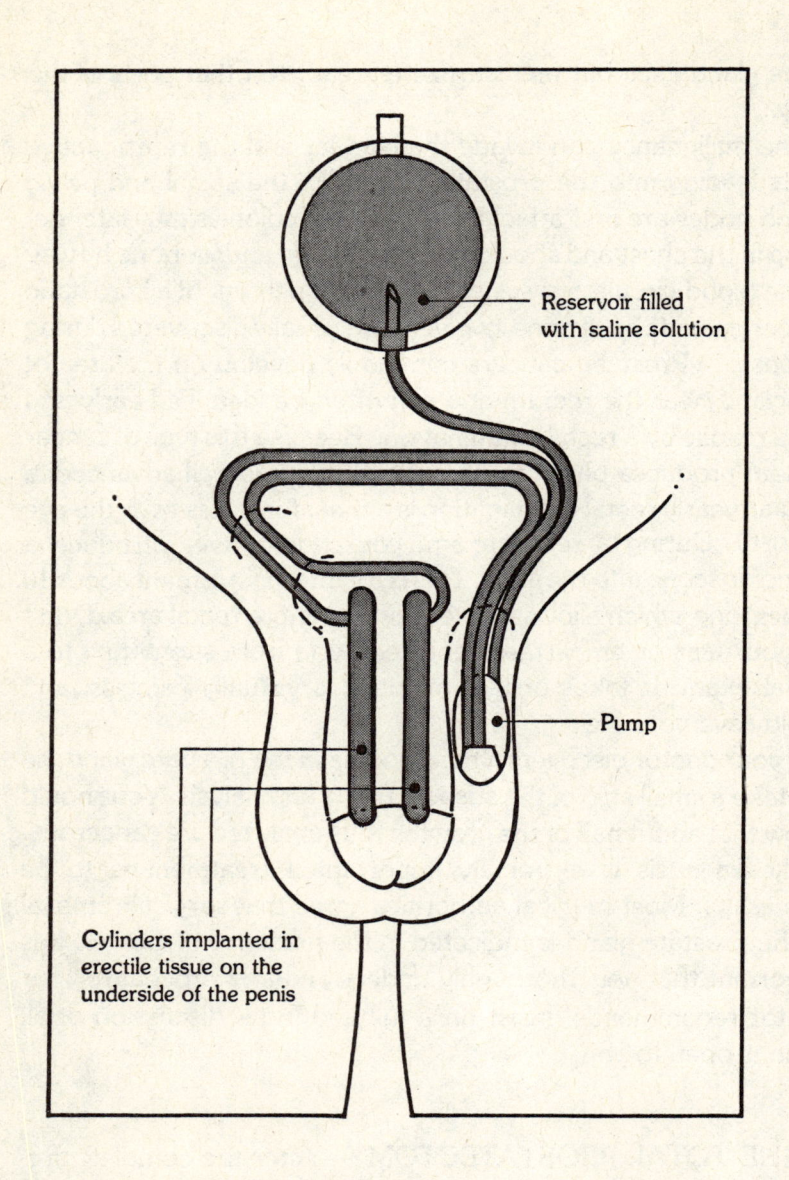

The Inflatable Penile Prosthesis

Although the desire for sex is reduced by the removal of the gland, it does not disappear. Unfortunately, impotence and the inability to have an erection must be expected to occur. But, through the miracles of modern technology, science has found a way to artificially create a perfectly respectable erection whenever the need arises. Males must certainly not allow mistaken notions or strong "macho" ideas to influence their decision on whether to accept prostate surgery.

THE PENIS PROSTHESIS—Let us make one thing perfectly clear. *No*, you're not going to lose your penis in prostate surgery, but it won't respond to sexual arousal as it did when you were nineteen either. The *inflatable penile prosthesis* is a surgical implant inserted into the erectile tissue *(corpora cavernosa)* located on the back of the penis. This insert consists of two silicone rubber cylinders connected with tubing to a reservoir (filled with a sterile saline solution) on the abdominal wall. The tiny pump that works the device is implanted in the scrotum. *Implant* is the operative word here. All parts of this miraculous gizmo are implanted inside the body. Nothing shows on the outside.

When an erection is called for, a few squeezes on the pump inside the scrotum forces the saline solution into the ballon-like cylinders implanted in the penis. The penis responds by swelling in a near-normal manner and intercourse can proceed to the satisfaction of both partners.

After orgasm and ejaculation, a release valve on the pump is activated and the saline solution flows back into the reservoir. With a success rate of over 99 percent, studies have shown that both the male and his female partner approve the inflatable implant over the fixed-rod implant.

The *fixed-rod implant* consists of two semi-rigid silicone rods directly implanted in the penis. With this type of prosthesis, named the *Small-Carrion penile prosthesis* after its inventors, the male maintains a permanent semi-erection all the time. The disadvantages of this type of implant are obvious. It causes some very real physical discomfort and psychological strain. Males with the fixed-rod implant have reported they walk around with their hands in their pockets most of the time to disguise the fact that they have an uncontrolled erection.

An even better solution coming out of China is the news that Chinese surgeons have developed a method of constructing a new *flesh and blood penis* for men who have lost their natural organs. The official *Xinhua* news agency of Peking, China recently revealed that plastic surgeons have successfully constructed and placed 27 artificial penises on men who have lost their organ to cancer or a severe injury. The penises are built from the patients' arm tissues and are attached in a single operation. The report concluded with this statement: "The patients have all regained sexual functions after the operations, which have taken place since 1983. One has since fathered a child and the wife of another is pregnant."

A Look At The Natural Preventives

Although the written word cannot substitute fully for the advice of a qualified and concerned physician, there are some measures you can safely take which many believe can improve and maintain the health of your prostate and insure continued normal functioning for a lifetime. One way is to make sure your diet provides all the vital nutrients that science has determined are necessary for this important gland and the entire glandular system.

BEE POLLEN—We invite you to consider the fact that Noel Johnson, the 87-year old marathon runner, says, "Bee pollen restored my manhood when I was almost 80 years old." It would certainly be safe to assume that his prostate is alive and well and functioning efficiently after a long period of dormancy. Noel says it was bee pollen that conquered the impotence that kept him out of the mainstream of life for so many years. See *Bee Pollen* (Chapter 13).

Studies conducted at both the Nagasaki University School of Medicine in Japan and the Urological Unit of the University of Lund in Sweden determined that oral bee pollen therapy reduced the swelling and inflammation accompanying severe prostatitis in the men tested. Both research groups reported that the continual and regular use of bee pollen was what did the trick. No adverse side effects were observed in the men taking the two different bee pollen preparations. World-wide studies on the effects of bee pollen in the case of prostate involvement confirm these findings.

Along with the full complement of nutrients identified in bee pollen, it offers a high concentration of zinc and magnesium, both shown to be particularly important in maintaining a healthy prostate.

ZINC—For more than half a century, science has known that the fluid produced by a healthy, normal prostate gland contains a very high concentration of zinc. In two landmark studies, the Mt. Sinai Medical Center and the Cook County Hospital, both located in Chicago, Illinois, reported on research showing that males with chronic prostatitis and/or prostatic cancer had a deficiency of zinc.

Male with prostatitis showed an average of only 50 mmg of zinc per milliliter of prostate fluid, but males with a healthy prostate had an average level of 448 mmg zinc per milliliter of fluid—a whopping nine times higher than their suffering brothers.

In the control groups, more than one out of every three of the men tested had inadequate amounts of zinc in their prostate fluid, although they still appeared healthy. Does this mean that the one out of every three exhibiting low levels of zinc will develop a prostate problem later in life? Some authorities think so.

Of the 200 male patients suffering from prostatitis who were given zinc supplements, more than 70 percent reported their symptoms were relieved. Each patient received from 11 to 34 milligrams of zinc daily for a period of four months. Note: This is *not* a do-it-yourself prescription. Only a chemical analysis by a competent physician can determine the precise amount of zinc (or anything else) which may be lacking in your personal body chemistry.

SEEDS & NUTS—Seeds and nuts are incredibly potent live foods. They contain the blueprints for their species and have the ability to reproduce life. Raw, natural seeds and nuts (not the commercially-processed greasy, roasted and salted varieties) are a valuable addition to anybody's diet, but are especially important in overcoming a prostate problem. They not only contain high-quality proteins, plus zinc and magnesium, they also offer essential fatty acids in a wholesome unsaturated form that the body will appreciate. Raw seeds and nuts are a rich source of the essential fatty acid *lecithin*. See *Nutrition for a Healthy Heart* (Chapter 18). Of the seeds, pumpkin, sunflower, sesame, and squash seeds are considered excellent. Of the nuts, almonds rate highest in nutrient content.

The renowned German nutritionist, Dr. W. Devrient, favors pumpkin seeds above all others. Dr. Devrient says there's practically no incidence of prostate disorders in areas of the world where pumpkin seeds are consumed in abundance. He writes, "Only the plain people know the secret of pumpkin seeds, a secret handed down from father to son for generations. All know that pumpkin seeds preserve the prostate gland and thereby the male potency. They are an inexhaustible source of vigor offered by Mother Nature."

ESSENTIAL FATTY ACIDS—Unsaturated essential fatty acids are sometimes referred to as Vitamin F. The essential fats are *linoleic, linolenic,* and *arachidonic* acid and they must be obtained in the diet. Good natural sources of these important friendly fats are cold-processed, unrefined vegetable oils. The best of the oils is *linseed,* (See *Linseed Oil* Chapter 6) followed by sunflower and cod-liver oils. Wheat germ is another good source.

Science has determined that men require up to five times more fatty acids than do women. These essential fats help maintain elasticity and lubricate all cell tissues. They assist the entire glandular system and help reduce serum cholesterol levels in the body. As a supplement, up to five tablespoons daily may be added to the diet.

VITAMIN E—Vitamin E speeds healing throughout the entire body. Research indicates that the essential fatty acids are absorbed and assimilated more efficiently in the presence of Vitamin E.

GENERAL DIETARY GUIDELINES—Some nutritionists recommend that up to 60 percent of the daily diet be in uncooked form. A healthy diet composed mainly of fruits, raw vegetables, and salad greens can exert a powerful cleansing effect which benefits the entire body. Caffeinated beverages of all kinds (coffee, tea, soda) and alcohol should be avoided, as should overly spicy foods.

SUPPLEMENTS—Along with the bee pollen and zinc mentioned above, additional food supplements thought to be of assistance in maintaining prostate health include: Brewer's Yeast, Vitamin C, E, and F (essential fatty acids), and Chlorophyll.

The Botanical Medicinals

Although there is no substitute for competent medical advice and treatment in the case of prostate involvement, an adjunctive herbal therapy may help. Sounding more like a miracle than a treatment, a European herb has been reported as providing astounding results abroad in many cases of prostate problems. From published reports abroad, we bring you the following information.

THE SMALL-FLOWERED WILLOW HERB—A renowned German herbalist has recently revealed amazing case histories of prostatitis cures wrought by a little-known European herb. *Epilobium parviflorum,* the Small-Flowered Willow Herb, is a centuries-old remedy for diseases of the genito-urinary tract.

Although very few herbal books mention the Small-Flowered Willow Herb in any connection, the last known being in a herbal published as far back as 1880, this 'lost' herb is proving to be of great value in easing prostate problems and, at least in some cases, was so effective and healed so quickly that scheduled surgery was not necessary.

Before we go into a brief summary of these cases, it is necessary for you to understand that medicinal herbs are in widespread use in Europe and the Iron Curtain countries. The natural healing herbs are a respected and time-honored part of medical pharmacopeia abroad. We are not discussing 'witches and spells'; we are reporting on botanical substances which have been shown to ease and assist healing in certain conditions of ill health.

A case in point, as related in an important book called *Miracle Healing Power Through Nature's Pharmacy* (Fischer Publishing, Canfield, Ohio), is the story of Eric Johnson who wrote, "I beg you to show me a way back to health and give my family back their healthy father."

With a long history of inflammation of the prostate, Johnson had gone from one doctor to another seeking relief. He was in despair. He developed a duodenal ulcer and serious liver complications when all his friendly intestinal bacteria were destroyed by the strong medications he was taking. He passed pus and blood with every bowel movement.

Mr. Johnson became very ill and his doctor took him off all chemical medication. He was operated on, but still the inflammation did not clear up. Again, his physician put him on medication and gave him injections and again his condition worsened. He only began to improve when he began taking medicinal herbs regularly. All his years of suffering might have been avoided had he known of the Willow Herb earlier.

In another case, a man who recovered from a prostate disorder tells how the Willow Herb relieved his dysfunction. The unfortunate man, one Paul Soames, was in the hospital being treated for a serious heart infarction. Because of his heart condition, his physician felt he could not withstand an operation on his prostate.

He writes, "I heard of the wonderful Willow Herb which has helped in so many similar cases and began to drink an infusion (tea) daily. After several days, I had no more complaints and still drink the tea daily for a complete recovery. I thank God from the bottom of my heart. It is unbelievable that medicinal plants give such results!"

Another documented case concerns a European priest, a Father Homan, who suffered from terminal cancer of the prostate gland. When his doctors gave up, he turned to a natural healer who recommended the Willow Herb. We are pleased to be able to report that the good Father is once again able to continue with his religious works.

Although not related to the prostate, another story demonstrating the potency of the Willow Herb concerns a James McMillan, who had undergone three different operations for bladder cancer and who was in great pain. After taking Willow Herb tea for some months, he made a full recovery, which was verified by his astonished doctor.

PROSTASAN 7™—*Prostasan 7*, new to the U.S., is the original Hanne Kramb formula (See *Impotence*, Chapter 12) and is one of the preparations Hanne Kramb recommends for male impotence. It is now being produced in the U.S. especially for the American market by BioLife Pharmacals. This blend of important medicinal botanicals has been tallying up amazing success stories abroad. Prostasan 7 contains the maximum amount of the Small-Flowered Willow Herb, and is the precise formulation used so skillfully and successfully against common prostate problems by Hanne Kramb in two years of clinical testing in Germany.

Beginning with a healthy measure of the Small-Flowered Willow Herb, this healing remedy for a distressed prostate is fortified with Horsetail, Sage, and Saw Palmetto (Sabal serrulata) and is used by herbalists for its diuretic, stimulating, and tonic properties. This herb is considered valuable because of its ability to provide nutrition for the testicles in cases of atrophy. It has an historic reputation as a remedy for prostate disorders and male complaints of all kinds.

Prostasan 7 is provided in the form of a loose tea to facilitate the brewing of individualized strengths, as either a powerful preventive or potent medicinal.

Additional Herbal Helps

DAMIANA—In his work, *Materia Medica Vegetablis*, Steinmetz of Holland says the following of Damiana (Turnera aphrodisiaca): "The leaves are a stimulant in sexual weakness and a tonic to the nerves. This botanical overcomes exhaustion and is esteemed for its aphrodisiac properties and its excellent effect on the reproductive organ."

In the early 1900's, Dr. W.H. Myers, a U.S. physician, used Damiana extensively in his practice. He wrote, "I find that in cases of partial impotence or other sexual debility, Damiana's success is universal."

GINSENG—One of the most highly prized medicinals in the Chinese Pharmacopeia, Ginseng (Panax notoginseng) is said to stimulate production of hormones, thereby assisting the sex glands. This potent herb has been used for centuries. It is believed to rejuvenate the most debilitated and increase longevity.

Massaging The Prostate

The noted medical nutritionist and writer, Paavo Airola, developed an exercise specifically for prostate disorders. The directions for a self-manipulation and massage of the prostate can be found in many of his books, as follows:

The male is directed to lie flat on his back on a hard surface. Draw the knees upward toward the chest. Point the knees outward and press the soles of the feet together. While keeping the soles of the feet together, lower legs as far as possible and return. Repeat this movement with as much force as can be managed as many times per session as the patient can handle.

Note: It would be advisable for seniors especially (and beginners of any age) to solicit some help in assuming the position and completing the movements specified to make sure the exercise can be accomplished without strain.

Natural Biological Urges

There are many authorities who believe that it is unhealthy in the extreme for the male to attain a state of sexual arousal without the natural release of orgasm and ejaculation. Males who, for one reason or another, do not regularly engage in the sexual act may be setting themselves up for prostate problems later in life. A suppressed or incomplete ejaculation, and/or practicing withdrawal without orgasm as a form of primitive birth control, has been shown to be very risky. Science says that a prolonged engorgement of the penis without release can lead to functional and/or structural damage of the prostate.

Conclusion

As in all conditions of ill health, preventing a prostate problem is much easier than relying on medical treatment when one arises. Adding some high-quality nutrients and supplements to your diet is one easy way to insure continued prostate health. Also, specific medicinal botanicals have been shown useful in certain instances of prostate involvement. But by far the easiest prescription to follow is to enjoy a robust and healthy sex life for a lifetime.

CHAPTER 12

New Help & Hope For The Impotent

Cause & Effect

WHEN YOU CAN'T—No man has to be told what this means. The experts say that an occasional occurrence of impotence is really nothing to worry about. It can be caused by something as simple as imbibing too freely or being overtired. As a point of fact, there are times when the best of us can't.

Identifying the Cause of the Problem

Impotence is medically defined as "the inability of the male to copulate". Medical science identifies the condition in various terms by establishing the cause. *Anatomic* impotence is the name given to a defect in the genitalia. *Atonic* refers to a paralysis of the nerves that carry the impulses which stimulate an erection. *Functional* impotence (not due to an anatomical defect) is defined as of psychogenic (mental) origin. *Psychic* impotence is more serious and is identified as a mental disturbance. *Symptomatic* impotence is due to generally poor health (a lack of certain nutrients), the presence of disease, or may be the result of taking certain drugs.

For a very long time, many of us have believed that becoming impotent was something to be expected in the normal course of aging. But there are too many examples of strong virile men who maintain (or regain) their sexuality into their 80s and beyond for us to accept impotence as normal. The inspiring story of *Noel Johnson* (see Chapter 13) is a case in point.

And research has determined that, at least in certain instances, there are a number of factors contributing to impotence that we can very easily do something about right now.

Nutrient and Hormone Deficiencies

Poor physical condition plays a part in setting the stage for impotence. A chronic low-grade barely detectable infection, resulting in fatigue and apathy, is more common than generally supposed. Lack of sufficient exercise and an inadequate diet keep many males teetering on the verge of a real illness.

It has been said that the United States is the best-fed but least-nourished nation in the world today. Commercially processed foods are loaded with chemical additives. Growth-hormones are fed to meat animals and poultry. Insecticides and fertilizers enter the food chain through agricultural crops. Many vitamins, minerals, and important nutrients are lost in the processing of the foods we put on the dinner table, and then put back in with artificial chemical compounds. Our foods are full of preservatives, stabilizers, and synthetic vitamins and minerals.

It's no wonder that the U.S. is declining yearly on the list of the world's healthiest countries. We are eating chemically processed, unnatural dead food with no enzyme activity. Is it any wonder that we have millions and millions of sick and unhealthy people in the richest country in the world?

BEE POLLEN—In the raw granular state, these golden grains from the beehive possess extraordinarily active enzymes, vital to so many internal processes of the body. If correctly cold-processed, the enzyme activity of the bee pollen remains in the finished product. Bee pollen contains all the vitamins, minerals, enzymes, hormones, proteins, carbohydrates, essential fatty acids, and trace elements identified as necessary in human nutrition.

Bee pollen contains one of the important elements vital to the subject of this chapter, a *gonadatropic* hormone. This plant hormone is very similar to the pituitary sex hormone, *gonadatropin*, which functions as a sex gland stimulant.

For a full discussion on bee pollen, including its documented benefits in overcoming impotence, please see "Bee Pollen" (Chapter 13).

Drugs as a Contributing Factor

MEDICATION—In a Minnesota study of approximately 200 impotent males, one of the largest contributing factors was discovered to be the medication the men were taking.

In this group, almost all were taking drugs to control high blood pressure (diuretics, antihypertensives, vasodilators). The onset of impotence closely coincided with the time the men began taking the drug.

Note: If impotence is a problem for you, you might want to backtrack and make a mental check of any medications you take regularly. Drugs other than antihypertensives implicated in the onset of impotence include medications prescribed for an ulcer or a psychiatric condition. Question your doctor if you suspect a relationship.

High Blood Pressure

Because many of the drugs commonly used to control high blood pressure have been shown to be a factor in the onset of impotence, let's take a brief look here at hypertension.

The mechanisms which regulate blood pressure involve many

body organs, hormones, and nerve impulses. Because any irregularity arising within this complicated network may create hypertension, detecting the exact cause is very difficult, but certain high risk factors have been identified, including:

Stress: One of the effects of continued stress is a serious elevation of blood pressure.

Sodium: Excessive intake of salt increases blood pressure.

Drugs: Some medications (even simple decongestants) can cause blood pressure to rise.

Weight: Carrying excess weight is usually accompanied by a rise in blood pressure, especially between the ages of 24 and 36.

Tobacco: Smoking has been tied to both heart disease and cancer, as well as a sharp rise in blood pressure.

Heredity: If one or both parents have high blood pressure, the children of that union will most likely develop the condition.

When you read through this list of increased risk factors - *did you recognize that you can control every single one of them -* except the last?

DIAGNOSING HYPERTENSION—High blood pressure, often called the 'silent killer,' rarely produces definitive symptoms. Some hypertensive individuals complain of headaches, stress, shortness of breath, dizziness, and feeling tired, but others feel very well. This fact alone demonstrates the need for regular checkups.

The stress of a visit to your doctor's office very often temporarily raises your blood pressure. If your blood pressure reading should fall in the high range, don't begin worrying needlessly. At least three separate high readings are required before a careful doctor will make a definite diagnosis.

Science has also determined that the cardiovascular system can satisfactorily adjust to high blood pressure for a period of time. However, long-term hypertension can lead to heart and kidney damage and eventually even the eyes and brain are affected.

Once a diagnosis of hypertension has been made, you may have to take medication for life. But life is still sweet and high blood pressure can be controlled by following your doctor's orders and making some changes in your lifestyle.

HELP YOURSELF—Along with making some obvious changes in your diet, such as watching your intake of salt and losing excess weight, have your blood pressure monitored regularly, *and*

Shun tobacco. Give up cigarettes, cigars, and that pipe you think makes you look so distinguished, *and*

Question your doctor about any medications (over-the-counter and/or prescription drugs) you take to determine if they are involved in any increase in your blood pressure, *and*

EXERCISE—Authorities agree that exercising (aerobic) just three times per week for around 30 minutes can reduce hypertension. See *Rebounding* (Chapter 1). The Institute for Aerobics Research (Dallas, Texas) recently completed a study which proves this hypothesis: After a walk-jog program lasting just four months, the subjects had reduced their systolic pressure an average of 12 points and their diastolic pressure 7 points.

Exercise regularly, *and*

CHECK YOUR DIET—*Fats:* Simply cutting back on saturated fats has been shown to help in lowering blood pressure. See *Linseed Oil* (Chapter 6). Cutting down on fats assists in weight loss, too.

Meats: Switching to a vegetarian diet reduces blood pressure because a meatless diet is low in salt, high in fiber, potassium, and polyunsaturated fats. If meat is your passion, eat less red meat and substitute skinned poultry and fish.

Calcium: Dairy products are the major source. Choose low-fat low-sodium varieties. Men need up to 1000 mg calcium daily.

Potassium: Increased intake helps the body to excrete the sodium (salt) which promotes fluid buildup. Fluid retention increases stress on the heart and entire circulatory system and is a major cause of high blood pressure.

Fruits: With their high content of Vitamin C and important bioflavonoids See *Vitamin P* (Chapter 3). Fresh citrus strengthens blood vessels and capillaries. Bioflavonoids (Vitamin P) are in the white membranes separating the sections and are lost in juicing. Enjoy your fruit whole, *and*

REFUSE STRESS—Please note that we are not suggesting that you 'avoid' stress. Stress is part and parcel of living — and always has been. It's not a 'modern' invention at all. Consider the caveman stalking a ferocious wild beast to feed his family and count your blessings.

There are many relaxation techniques (biofeedback, meditation) aimed at controlling stress and which have been shown to reduce hypertension. If stress is a part of your life, you can deal with the situation and then refuse to allow it to affect you. Take a walk (or a vacation), play with the kids (or the dog), practice deep breathing (or go deepsea fishing). Learn to 'go with the flow' and relax! See *Conquering Depression and Handling Stress* (Chapter 19).

Does it seem that we are straying far afield from the subject of this chapter? Not at all. If antihypertensive drugs contribute to impotence (and studies agree that they do), making some healthy changes in your lifestyle can reduce high blood pressure (if you have it), and these same healthy changes are documented preventives as well. Maintaining normal blood pressure means that you won't have to take (possible impotence inducing) drugs to control high blood pressure levels and this contributing factor is thus avoided.

Note: We are in no way suggesting that you discontinue taking high blood pressure medication as prescribed by your doctor. Hypertension is a life-threatening condition and it must be controlled.

Impaired Circulation

POOR CIRCULATION—In the 1940s, the well-known Kinsey Report documented an increase in male impotence after the age of 50, a strong argument in favor of aging as a factor. But irrefutable data also shows that the incidence of atherosclerosis is higher after the half-century mark. Atherosclerosis is primarily a circulatory problem arising because deposits of arteriosclerotic plaque in blood vessels have narrowed the passageways.

A recent French study has observed that a free-flowing supply of blood is needed to achieve an erection. *Voila!* The wonder is that it took so long to make this common-sense connection between the inability to achieve an erection and circulation. Obviously, clogged-up arteries (frequent, remember, after the age of 50), cannot supply the powerful surge of blood needed to engorge the erectal tissue of the penis. The result is a weak erection or none at all.

In an examination of approximately 450 impotent males, the French scientists tabulated the factors known to contribute to impaired circulation (smoking, diabetes, high blood pressure, high cholesterol and triglyceride levels).

Over 90 percent of the impotent males over 40 examined by the French researchers had one or two of these factors working against them. The report concluded, "The increase in the frequency of impotence with age is mainly related to arteriosclerotic changes in the arteries which supply the penis. The arterial risk factors should be evaluated in any patient complaining of impotence."

THE F-M CIRCULIZER SYSTEM—Because one of the major causes of impotence certainly has to be impaired circulation, this circulation stimulating device from Europe may well prove to be of invaluable help. First introduced in *Miracle Healing Power Through Nature's Pharmacy* (Fischer Publishing, Canfield, Ohio), this device is still not widely known in the U.S. For complete information on the benefits of this revolutionary therapeutic system from across the ocean, please see Chapter 10.

OTHER WAYS TO IMPROVE CIRCULATION—Reducing saturated fats in the diet is documented to assist in reducing unhealthy cholesterol and triglyceride levels related to the development of arteriosclerotic plaque. (See *Linseed Oil*, Chapter 6). Regular aerobic exercise both stimulates blood flow and strengthens veins and arteries. (See *Rebounding*, Chapter 1). Bioflavonoids aid distressed capillaries (the tiniest blood vessels) and help the entire circulatory system. (See *Vitamin P*, Chapter 3).

Introducing Hanne Kramb

Although she is often called "The Miracle Lady of Honzrath," Hanne Kramb (of the renowned Hanne Kramb Clinic in West Germany), rejects that honorific title. In the spring of 1986, I spent a great deal of time with the great lady and have to confess to being very impressed. This 50-year old dynamo works her miracles in a matter-of-fact no-nonsense manner. I personally witnessed some really astounding healings and feel very privileged to have been let in on a few of her secrets.

Hanne Kramb treats a wide range of diseases and conditions of ill health. While I was waiting for her one very cold morning, I struck up a conversation with an elderly woman who had suffered for many years with Parkinson's diseases. She cheerfully told me that just a few months before entering the Hanne Kramb Clinic, she shook so violently that she was unable to feed herself. I marveled at this tiny lady. She exhibited no sign of the palsy and tremors that are a mark of this condition.

IMPOTENCE—I also learned that Hanne Kramb has accomplished an incredible advancement in the treatment of male sexual dysfunction. This justly renowned German physician has had such a miraculous rate of success in regenerating and rejuvenating impotent males (of any age) and returning them to full vigor and virility that she positively guarantees a cure.

From America to Zanzibar (and everywhere in between), a constant stream of health seekers visits her clinic. Everyone from heads-of-state to well-known Hollywood personalities to little-known executives of international corporations to common folk (just like you and me) come knocking on her door.

Confidentiality is paramount and no names are ever revealed, but one gentleman of over sixty-five years told me proudly that his considerably younger wife had no complaints. He confided to me that their relationship had begun while she was working as his secretary. Over a four-year period, they gradually realized that they loved one another. When his wife of many years died, he began taking her out for little dinners and they became very close. But when she talked of a future together, he resisted and confessed to her that he was impotent. It was only after taking Hanne Kramb's course of treatment that they were married. Apparently, this June-November marriage is very happy.

Another man I talked to was only around forty years old. He was more reticent and I never got the details of his case, but he did let slip that he was being treated by Hanne Kramb for impotence. He smiled constantly and looked very relaxed, so my guess is that she was successful once again.

The 'catch', of course, is that it's necessary to visit her West German clinic and take the full three-week course of treatment. To conquer impotence, Hanne Kramb uses a combination of acupuncture, intravenous injections of certain natural substances, and the oral administration of special capsules containing her personal secret formula. Hanne Kramb's capsules, potent as they are, cannot do the work alone. Because this is a combination therapy, each element of the treatment works in conjuction with the others. It is for this reason that she requires the presence of the patient. I feel the need to stress here that Hanne Kramb could probably make a lot of money by offering her capsules (alone) for sale by mail order. She rejects this approach without equivocation, explaining that money and personal wealth are not her primary motivation. This doctor genuinely wants to heal. The cost of Hanne Kramb's guaranteed impotence cure amounts to approximately $3,500.00. This fee includes accomodations and meals for the entire length of the three-week treatment, but not airfare. As a courtesy, she will extend a five percent discount off the total amount of this revolutionary therapy to readers of the expanded and revised *Hidden Secrets of Super-Perfect Health* that you hold in your hand. I recognize that, even after taking the five percent discount, this is a costly treatment. However, if you are an impotent male, you are the only one who can decide if a guaranteed cure is worth this expense. Hanne Kramb regrets that she is unable to reply directly to any inquiries.

For more information on Hanne Kramb's treatment contact New Dimensions Distributors listed at the back of this book.

*Noel Johnson—87 Year Old Marathon Runner
What's his secret?*

Bee Pollen

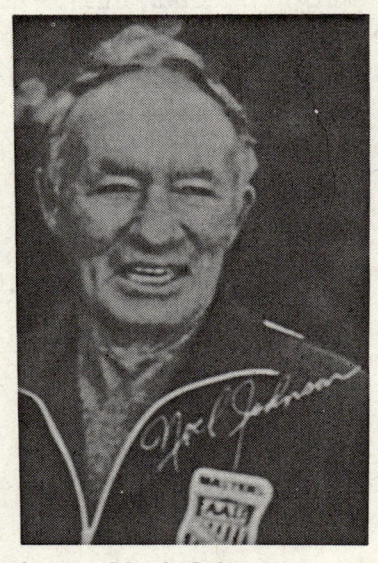

At 84 years of age, Noel Johnson was honored with the *President's Council on Physical Fitness & Sports Award.* The President's Council believes Johnson's healthy lifestyle is precisely the example millions of Americans need. Now 87, Noel competes in marathons around the world and has the gold medals to prove it. He holds the World's Senior Boxing Championship, often fighting men 30 years his junior to keep it. In 1984, he visited both Japan and Iceland lecturing, running and promoting his autobiography, which has been translated into both languages. In 1985, Noel Johnson applied to be the first octogenarian in space!

He has been recommended to NASA and just might end up being the world's oldest space cadet on some future space flight.

CHAPTER 13

Noel Johnson

The 87-Year Old Superman - A Profile

When Noel Johnson was born in the last century (July, 1899), he never dreamed of the fame that would come to him in the autumn of his life. He married, moved from his birthplace in Minnesota to California, fathered two children, and worked until his retirement at age 65 - just like millions of other Americans across our great land.

In his autobiography (published in 1982 by The Plains Corporation), Noel himself talked about his typical lifestyle in these words, "The hospitable Californians gathered us in and soon we were embarked on a round of parties and cookouts on the beach. It was all great fun and we ate and drank with the best of 'em. Even the birth of our two children didn't slow us down much. We figured life couldn't get much better than this. Pretty ordinary stuff, right?"

What is it, then, that sets this remarkable man apart from the great majority of us? Why has he been honored by President Ronald Reagan? Why do the officials of many nations around the world seek him out and fly him thousands of miles across huge oceans to their homelands to pay him homage and ask his counsel? Why do tremendous crowds gather wherever he appears to celebrate the very fact of his life? As a matter of fact, Noel is far from ordinary.

By his 70th birthday, Noel's whole life had changed. He was in dangerously poor health; his wife had died, and the only joy he had in his life was his great-grandsons. He says now that the free and easy lifestyle he had followed all his years was the largest single factor contributing to his decline. "After I retired and my wife Zola died, I just shuffled around the house," he explains. "I drank a lot of beer and ate whatever came to hand, mostly manufactured junk-food. Even the close relationship I had with my son and daughter and their families wasn't enough to bring me out of my deep funk."

"My doctor told me I had a serious heart condition and restricted any physical activity. He said I didn't even dare mow the lawn, saying I might not live to trim the borders. It sure was easy to follow his orders. I just didn't much care about anything. I realize now I was simply waiting for the next and final stop on the journey we call life. I figured that I had lived my Biblical three-score years and ten. In the traditional and conventional sense, my life was over. I was living alone, eating improperly, and deteriorating daily."

What happened next shook Noel to the core. His son proposed that he go into a nursing home, saying that he needed someone to look after him properly. Noel sat himself down and, for the first time in a long time, began to think - hard! He analyzed his physical condition very harshly and discovered he was 40 pounds overweight, putting a strain on his already damaged heart.

"I had all the classic signs of aging and ill-health," he says. "Bulging gut, lackluster eyes. My unused muscles hung slack. I looked defeated. But I used to be a boxer and the thought "defeated" stirred something in my ego. I decided then and there to beat the bell and come out swinging. They can't count you out when you're trying!"

What happened after that is history. Using a program of good natural foods, with bee pollen his secret weapon in the fight to regain his health, Noel began a gradually escalating program of exercise fueled with bee pollen and deep determination.

Noel says, "I made honeybee pollen the one unvarying and

essential foundation of my rejuvenation program. Since I discovered bee pollen at the age of 70, this perfect live food has restored my manhood, brought me physically to full vigor, and continues to nourish every cell in my body while also protecting my health. I am simply never sick. I made it...and you can, too!"

There is no doubt whatsoever that Noel has 'made it.' This incredible man competes in marathon runs of 26-plus miles around the world and has the gold medals to prove it! He has been named "superman" by doctors who delight in studying him to find out how he has so successfully reversed the aging process. He is a favorite guest on important talk shows, and interviews with Noel have been featured in many popular magazines, newspapers, and other publications. He appeared on five million Wheaties boxes in 1977 in their "Breakfast of Champions" series and was recently approached again by the Wheaties people. They want to do another five million boxes showing this dynamite champion in 1986! Some snapshots from Noel's personal photo album follow.

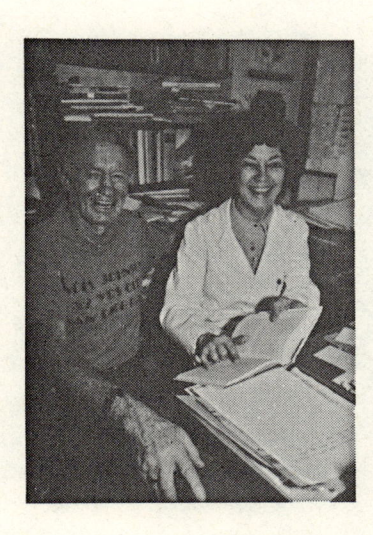

Today, at 87 years of age, the doctors who have examined me trying to find out how I've reversed the aging process, call me "superman."

At left, with Dr. Lenora Zohman, a respected cardiologist, Dr. Zohman is explaining the forthcoming tests to me.

162 / *Hidden Secrets of Super-Perfect Health*

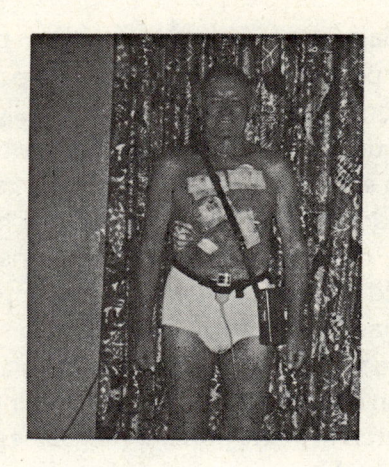

Trying to find out what makes 'superman' tick

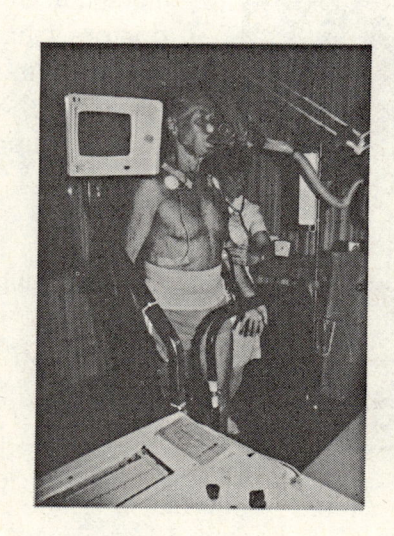

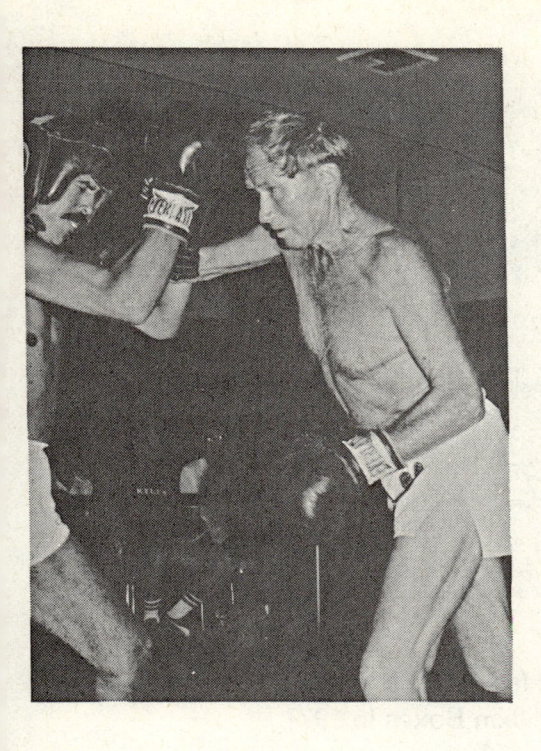

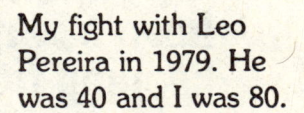

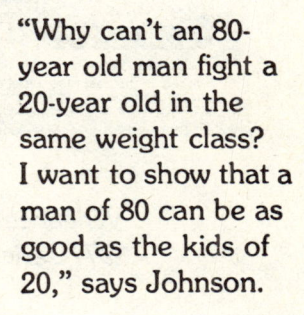

My fight with Leo Pereira in 1979. He was 40 and I was 80.

"Why can't an 80-year old man fight a 20-year old in the same weight class? I want to show that a man of 80 can be as good as the kids of 20," says Johnson.

Last July he won his fifth straight title in the 101th annual Senior Olympics Boxing Championship in Los Angeles, defeating his 40-year old opponent.

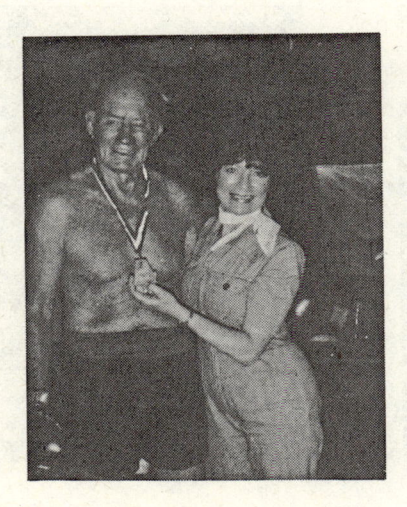

Sybil Jason presenting me with the gold medal after the fight.

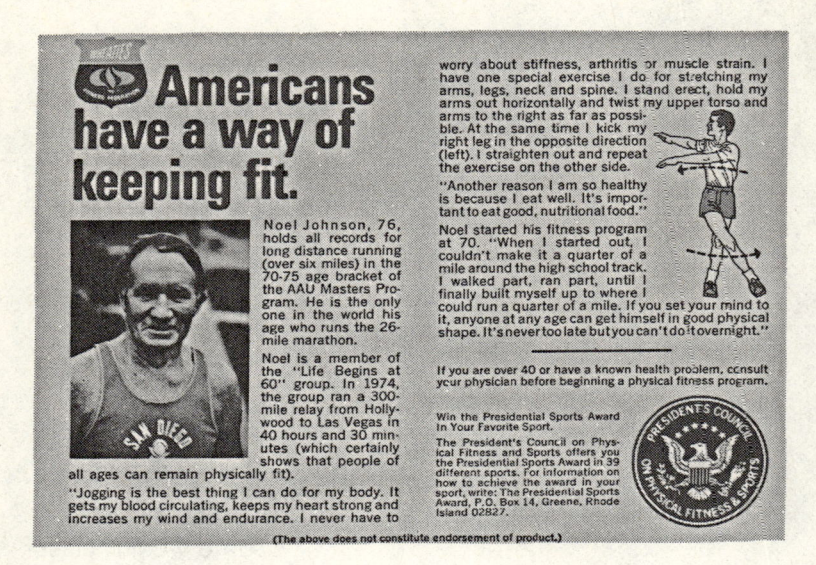

164 / Hidden Secrets of Super-Perfect Health

Americans have a way of keeping fit.

Noel Johnson, 76, holds all records for long distance running (over six miles) in the 70-75 age bracket of the AAU Masters Program. He is the only one in the world his age who runs the 26-mile marathon.

Noel is a member of the "Life Begins at 60" group. In 1974, the group ran a 300-mile relay from Hollywood to Las Vegas in 40 hours and 30 minutes (which certainly shows that people of all ages can remain physically fit).

"Jogging is the best thing I can do for my body. It gets my blood circulating, keeps my heart strong and increases my wind and endurance. I never have to worry about stiffness, arthritis or muscle strain. I have one special exercise I do for stretching my arms, legs, neck and spine. I stand erect, hold my arms out horizontally and twist my upper torso and arms to the right as far as possible. At the same time I kick my right leg in the opposite direction (left). I straighten out and repeat the exercise on the other side.

"Another reason I am so healthy is because I eat well. It's important to eat good, nutritional food."

Noel started his fitness program at 70. "When I started out, I couldn't make it a quarter of a mile around the high school track. I walked part, ran part, until I finally built myself up to where I could run a quarter of a mile. If you set your mind to it, anyone at any age can get himself in good physical shape. It's never too late but you can't do it overnight."

If you are over 40 or have a known health problem, consult your physician before beginning a physical fitness program.

Win the Presidential Sports Award in Your Favorite Sport.

The President's Council on Physical Fitness and Sports offers you the Presidential Sports Award in 39 different sports. For information on how to achieve the award in your sport, write: The Presidential Sports Award, P.O. Box 14, Greene, Rhode Island 02827.

(The above does not constitute endorsement of product.)

Wheaties "Breakfast of Champions"
1977 series - 5 Million Boxes in 1977.

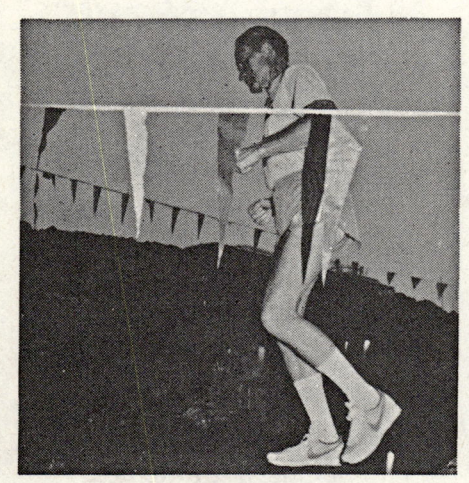

Pike's Peak -
14,000 feet straight UP
Noel Crossing the Finish Line

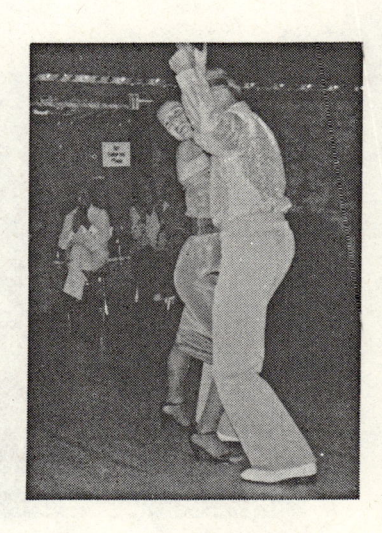

Saturday Night Fever!

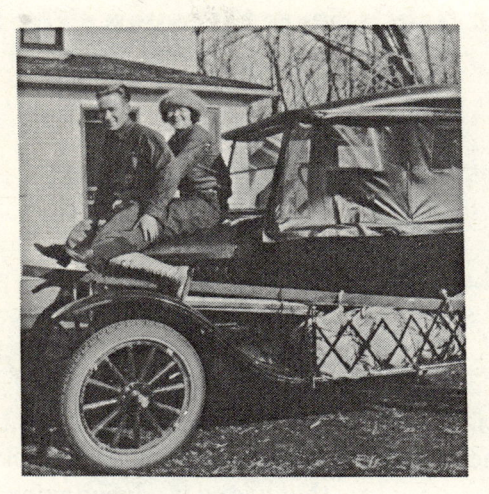

Noel & Zola - November 1923

Johnson says, "I'll be in better condition at age 90 than I am today! I know what you have to do to rebuild and keep your cells alive and I know what causes illness!"

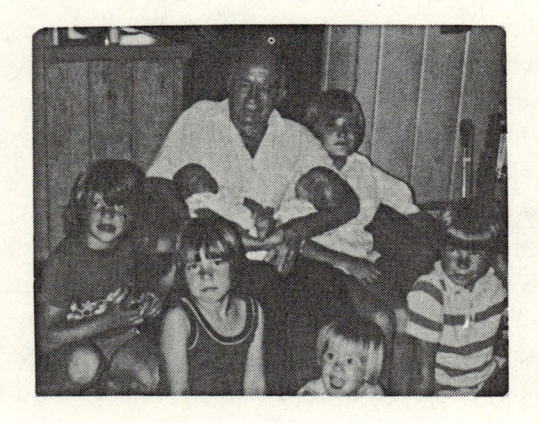

Noel today with his 7 Great-Grandsons

Analyzing Noel's Secret Weapon - The Mighty Bee Pollen

These Golden Grains Pack A Potent Punch

One of the most interesting things about bee pollen is that it *cannot be synthesized in a laboratory*. Oh yes, bee pollen contains all the vitamins, minerals, amino acids (proteins), hormones, enzymes, carbohydrates, essential fatty acids, and trace elements known to be needed in human nutrition. But as if that were not enough, Mother Nature (personified by the bee) adds a mysterious extra that has so far defied scientific analysis. In fact, some researchers believe it's this mysterious unidentifiable extra constituent which makes bee pollen the undeniably powerhouse nutrition that it is. It's important to note here that pollen collected mechanically directly from plants (sometimes called 'flower pollen') without the intervention of the bee is without this important extra factor.

Another one of nature's little mysteries is the fact that bee pollen contains a live electric charge. Dr. Eric H. Erickson, of the University of Wisconsin's Entomology Department, reports that when the worker bees leave the hive, they have a slightly negative or neutral electrical charge. But, upon returning to the hive with their pollen baskets loaded, the same bees register a positive charge of electricity as great as 1.5 volts! The live energized bee pollen they carry is also electrically charged.

Just what is this incredible natural substance? Pollen is the live male spore of all botanicals and is necessary for fertilization and growth of the species. Each microscopically tiny speck of this golden dust has the ability to reproduce. Bees unerringly select only the most powerful and potent pollens as food for the hive, another reason why bee pollen is superior to mechanically-collected pollen. Bee larvae, young bees, and the Queen eat only royal jelly.

Examining The Evidence

INCREASING THE LIFE SPAN—Who says so? Noel Johnson and U.S. President Ronald Reagan (now 73 and a well-publicized proponent of bee pollen), are not the only ones who acknowledge the power of pollen to extend life expectancy beyond the norm.

The countries behind the Iron Curtain have published considerable research on the beneficial effects of this near-perfect food. Professor Nikolai V. Tsitsin, U.S.S.R. botanist and biologist, investigated the lifestyle of the centenarians past 125 years of age living in the Caucasus mountains of upper Russia. He reported that many were beekeepers and the villagers all ate the sticky residue found on the bottom of the hives as one of their principal foods.

On analyzing this mass, Tsitsin found it to be almost pure bee pollen. After intensive research, he determined that including bee pollen in their regular diet was responsible in a large part for the incredible age these people attained. Tsitsin was also impressed with the quality of their lives in that all these people were actively working and in singularly good health in spite of their advanced age.

Working independently, the same conclusions were reached by other U.S.S.R. scientists as well. Dr. Naum P. Yoirich of the Soviet Academy summarizes his research in these words, "Bee pollen is one of the original treasure-houses of nutrition and medicine. *Long lives are attained by bee pollen users.* It contains every important substance necessary to life."

Perhaps even more important for those of us discovering bee pollen late in life is the statement made by the Far East Institute of the Soviet Union in Vladivostok. These scientists concluded their research report by saying, *"Bee pollen has regenerative properties for the body. Bee pollen contains all the amino acids, mineral salts, vitamins, and enzymes in perfect proportion as needed by the organism."*

As a further demonstration of bee pollen's powerful regenerating and rejuvenating effect, consider a paper coming out of Sarajevo, Yugoslavia. In a well-publicized study, Yugoslav researchers at the University of Sarajevo used oral bee pollen therapy on a group of impotent men. After a thirty day period, over half were documented as showing an increase in the production of sperm, probably because bee pollen's gonadatropic hormones act as a reproductive-gland stimulant.

AN OVERVIEW OF THE BENEFITS OF BEE POLLEN— There has been so much material published in just the past five years on bee pollen that it's difficult to bring you a full and complete condensation of the many, many benefits this super-rich and incredibly nutritious food offers.

AS A STOREHOUSE OF NUTRIENTS - Because the important part that diet plays in keeping us well or making us sick has been well established, any food which has been demonstrated to contain every element the body requires has to qualify as a super-food. Laboratory analysis of bee pollen confirms that it contains all the health-promoting live nutrients the body needs to sustain life itself.

What's more, bee pollen, the super-food, delivers these nutrients in perfectly balanced proportions. And, isn't it nice to know that Mother Nature has packaged it so superbly? You really don't have to take laboratory chemicals with your breakfast in order to get all the vitamins and minerals you need daily.

Dr. Alain Callais, Academie d'Agriculture, Paris, informs us that bee pollen is richer in essential protein than any animal source and says it contains more amino acids than beef, meat, eggs, or cheese of equal weight.

MEDICALLY SPEAKING - Centuries ago, Hippocrates said, "Let your food be your medicine; Let your medicine be your food." As a medicinal food, bee pollen scores high points again.

As long ago as 1948, the Journal of the National Cancer Institute published results of a study conducted by Dr. William Robinson of the U.S.D.A. which determined that bee pollen contains an active anti-cancer element which has the power to slow the development of mammary tumors.

Dr. Peter Hernuss, a practicing oncologist (cancer specialist) at the University of Vienna, reported a "noticeable decrease in the side-effects of radiation therapy" on women with uterine cancer when bee pollen was added to their diet. Hair loss, nausea and vomiting, loss of appetite, bladder and rectal inflammations, were greatly reduced in the women who took bee pollen during the course of their radiation therapy.

A German/Swiss team of urologists reported that bee pollen ingestion proved most successful as a treatment of prostatitis and prevented the need for surgery in their study of over 170 men.

French scientists (Dr. Remy Chauvin, the Institute of Bee Culture, Paris, and Dr. E. Lenormand, the Paris Child Preventatorium) report that bee pollen contains an extremely active natural antibiotic able to correct a malfunction of the gastro-intestinal tract by destroying harmful bacteria.

British scientist Dr. G. J. Binding says, "Honeybee pollen provides an increased resistance to infection. It is a giant germ-killer in whose presence bacteria simply cannot exist."

In his popular book, *About Pollen,* author Carlson Wade sums it all up by saying, "The healing, rejuvenating and disease-fighting effects of this total nutrient are hard to believe, yet are fully documented. Aging, digestive upsets, prostate disease, sore throats, acne, fatigue, sexual problems, allergies, and a host of other problems have been successfully treated by the use of bee pollen."

WORLD-CLASS ATHLETES - Lasse Viren, the Finnish runner who took the gold in the 5000 and 10,000 meter events in both the 1972 and 1976 Olympic games says his speed and endurance come from bee pollen. The renowned Finnish coach, Antti Lananake, concurs. "Our studies," he says, "show bee pollen significantly improves the team's performance. Most of our athletes take a bee pollen food supplement."

Of all the running champions, the most famous quote of all comes from Steve Riddick, long called the "fastest man in the world." Riddick himself says, "After just two months on bee pollen, I felt as if my body shifted into a more powerful gear."

It took former U.S.S.R. Olympic track coach Remi Korchemny, now with the Pratt Institute in New York to provide the answers. Korchemny mounted a two-year double-blind study with Pratt athletes, giving some bee pollen and some a placebo. His conclusions proved beyond doubt that bee pollen increased their crucial recovery time after stressed performance and enabled the athletes taking bee pollen to actually improve their performance the second time around.

Noel Johnson, running marathons at age 87, and enjoying what he calls his "second lifetime" with the verve and zest of a young man, agrees.

Choosing The Right Bee Pollen

How do we secure this potent rejuvenating and health-giving miracle food for ourselves? Bee pollen is harvested directly from the hive by means of a pollen-trap fitted with a smooth wire screen. In order to enter the hive, the worker bee must pass through the wire screen which gently brushes off a portion of the pollen she has collected in her travels from flower to flower. This pollen then falls a few inches into a pollen drawer. The beekeeper periodically empties the drawer of its precious contents and *should* (some don't) refrigerate or freeze it to insure ultimate quality and freshness. When he has amassed a sufficient quantity, the beekeeper sells his bee pollen to one of several U.S. manufacturers for cleaning, processing, and packaging into product form.

We want to say a word here about quality bee pollens. If bee pollen is bee pollen, why not purchase the lowest priced product available? Well, my friends, while a rose by any other name may still smell as sweet, that premise does not apply when selecting a bee pollen source. There are good bee pollens that deliver a full measure of benefits and there are poor bee pollens. No matter what end product the manufacturer turns out, that product can only be as good as the bee pollen and other ingredients that went into its manufacture.

For instance, when you find bee pollen granules that are as hard as pebbles, you may be sure that they have been overdried at a heat high enough to destroy all the vital enzymatic action and reduce the nutrient value. You can easily apply this test yourself when purchasing bee pollen in granular form, but what about a capsulized or tableted product? It's very easy for a manufacturer to start with the cheapest grade Spanish pollen, for example. Once the product has been processed into capsules or tablets, there's just no way to determine what bee pollen has been used as its base ingredient.

Therefore, it's very important that you know and can trust the source of your bee pollen. By all means, shun all foreign products, some of which have been contaminated with carbon tetrachloride, most of which are heated, and all of which are old by the time they reach our shores.

In judging only the U.S. packagers of raw granules, there's more than one good brand available. Touted as being from the clean, sunwashed high mountains and deserts of the western states, one of the newest and best is *Desert Gold*™ from BioLife Pharmacals. BioLife purchases their raw product from the same source as does C C Pollen Company, the producers of *High-Desert*®. Another excellent source of granules is The Montana Pollen & Herb Company, packaging under the well-known name of *Montana Big Sky*™.

These companies supply a very high grade of blended bee pollens gathered exclusively in the clean mountains and high desert areas of the western United States. Because no single-source pollen can supply a full complement of nutrients, a multi-source blend of bee pollens becomes obviously very important. In addition, these golden grains are harvested far from the environmental pollution that drifts over the cities, streets, and even the farms of the nation, assuring you fresh, pure, uncontaminated bee pollen with all the goodness Mother Nature intended packed into each tiny granule. In fact, the virgin high deserts and mountains of the United States might just be some of the few places left in the world where man has not intruded with chemical fertilizers, insecticides, and other pollutants.

In addition, any excess moisture found in these harvests is removed with an exclusive cold process at around 70 degrees. Testing reveals that each golden grain delivered by BioLife (*Desert Gold*™), Montana Pollen & Herb (*Montana Big Sky*™), and the C C Pollen Company is fully enzyme active.

Note: Pollens collected in many areas require the application of heat to preserve them from molding. Excessive heat destroys the live, vital nutrients that Mother Nature has so neatly packed into each tiny granule and kills the vital enzyme activity, resulting in a 'dead' food.

If you prefer the convenience of a premeasured dose, a powerful bee pollen product in an incredibly potent and unique new formulation is being sold under the trademarked name of *Bee Pollesan Gold*™. Each capsule contains top quality bee pollen, Siberian Ginseng, and the herb Gotu kola, all integrated into a base of pure Royal Jelly. These additional ingredients both potentiate and synergistically increase the activity of the bee pollen, as well as providing important benefits of their own.

To show you exactly *why* we believe *Bee Pollesan Gold* is the best bee pollen combination product available, let's examine the active principles of each of the additional ingredients separately without regard to the bee pollen itself.

Royal Jelly - Royal jelly is called the 'rejuvenation factor,' and with very good reason. Science now recognizes the power of royal jelly to transform a single larvae (identical in every way to her sister larva) into the royalty of the hive, the Queen Bee. Just exactly how this mysterious nutrient accomplishes this miracle is still unknown, but it is a documented fact that the Queen Bee lives for up to *five years*, while the worker bees of the hive have a lifespan of mere weeks. The only difference between the two is that the Queen alone feasts on royal jelly for the whole of her extended lifespan.

Can royal jelly work this same miracle in man? Research coming out of the U.S.S.R. confirms that royal jelly contains *acetylcholine,* an important element shown on autopsy to be lacking in the brains of Alzheimer's Disease victims. The Soviet findings also state that royal jelly regulates blood pressure, stimulates the suprarenal glands, enhances the immune system, is effective in cases of arteriosclerosis and coronary deficiency, reduces cholesterol, and restores energy where it is lacking.

Siberian Ginseng - In contrast to the more common Korean ginseng (grown strictly for the lucrative commercial market in worn out fields), Siberian ginseng (*Eleutherococcus*) is expensive, but worth it. It is biologically active, very potent, and possesses all the properties that have made ginseng sought after for centuries.

In the traditional Chinese pharmacopeia of medicines, ginseng is known as the cure-all herb. It contains Vitamins A, B12, and E, plus thiamine, riboflavin, niacin, calcium, iron, phosphorus, potassium, magnesium, and sulphur. Ginseng is used in the Orient to overcome stress, to stimulate and improve brain function, as an antidote to drugs and toxins, to normalize blood pressure, reduce harmful cholesterol levels, and to energize and generally enhance health. Ginseng is considered a powerful youth restorer and is said to inhibit the aging process itself. As a preventive, this 'King of Herbs' has no peer.

Gotu Kola—Gotu Kola (Hydrocotyle asiatica) is a natural herb that comes to us from the exotic islands of the Indian Ocean where the native doctors believe it contains remarkable stimulating and rejuvenating properties similar to those of ginseng (see above). An ancient Singhalese proverb says of Gotu Kola, "Eat two leaves a day to keep old age away." It contains Vitamins A, G, and K, and is rich in magnesium, plus small amounts of Vitamins E and B, and certain minerals. Herbologists use Gotu

Kola as a blood purifier, to fight physical and mental fatigue, and as a senility preventive.

NOTE: All the bee pollen products mentioned in this chapter are available in major health food stores nationwide, or may be ordered by mail direct from the distributor. Please see the final chapter for ordering information.

The Swiss Energy Formula

Bee pollen in particular is one of the nutrients acknowledged by the medical scientists of the world community of nations to be a powerful energizer, but it's not the only one. It seems appropriate to bring to your attention here another potent potion that is garnering high praise far and wide for its formula of nature's own nutrients as well.

BIO-STRATH - In the early 1950s, a physician by the name of Dr. Walther Strathmeyer and his patient, a Swiss victim of Meniere's disorder by the name of Fred Pestalozzi, made history when Pestalozzi was completely cured of his condition. What was this near-miraculous treatment that worked for Pestalozzi when everything else had failed? It was Dr. Strathmeyer's potent combination of all natural nutrients synergistically potentiated with the addition of a secret combination of wild herbs gathered from the clean, windswept Swiss mountainsides.

In the thirty-plus intervening years, Dr. Strathmeyer's powerful natural formula, *Bio-Strath*, has benefited millions. This product has been tested over and over again against various conditions by the meticulous Swiss, resulting in a body of enviable clinical documentation. Bio-Strath is currently imported from Switzerland by over thirty countries, the U.S. among them.

THE FORMULA - Bio-Strath is an easily assimilated liquid produced from a concentrated *Candida utilis* yeast strain and special wild herbs. For those who recognize the super-nutrition of yeast, but worry about the possibility of yeast infections, let us put your mind at rest immediately. The vaginitis which affects so many women (and men), commonly called a 'yeast infection,' is fed by *Candida albicans*, not *Candida utilis*. The pure nutritive yeast strain used in Bio-Strath comes from ripe, wild fruit. This special yeast is nutritionally active, but reproductively dormant. We emphasize that Bio-Strath does not, indeed *cannot*, contribute to any so-called 'yeast infection.'

Each batch of Bio-Strath requires two months to come to maturity. The Bio-Strath formula comes strictly from nature and is not produced from chemicals man-made in a laboratory. The result is a pleasant tasting nutritive-rich dietary supplement containing the special strain of yeast, wild herbs, malt, honey, and orange juice. What could be more natural?

Bio-Strath contains ten B-Complex vitamins, nineteen important minerals, eighteen amino acids (proteins), and nine active enzymes (necessary for assimilation and digestion), and is rich in RNA and DNA. The special *Candida utilis* yeast strain used in Bio-Strath consistently tests between two to four times higher in ATP (necessary for efficient cell functioning) than other yeasts. The Swiss allow no artificial colors, sweeteners, or preservatives to taint the pureness of Bio-Strath.

RESEARCH FINDINGS - The careful Swiss Health Authorities have recognized and licensed the production of all-natural Bio-Strath. In over twenty years of research and testing by independent laboratories, it has been demonstrated that Bio-Strath combats fatigue, nervousness, and lack of concentration. It increases both mental and physical efficiency, promotes vitality, and acts to provide an overall sense of well being to the organism. Even more important, Bio-Strath supports the immune system and builds resistence to disease.

WHO SAYS SO? - It is true that health authorities all over the world sing the praises of Bio-Strath. In the U.S., two medical doctors whose names are instantly recognizible to the majority of us have both gone public with their endorsement of this natural Swiss formula. Who are they?

Robert S. Mendelsohn, M.D. - Dr. Mendelsohn writes an enormously popular syndicated column, is a lecturer and author of note, and maintains a busy medical practice as well. It's important to stress here that Dr Mendelsohn has been approached many times by companies eager to secure his endorsement and has always refused - until now. Bio-Strath is the first and only product he has ever endorsed. In his own words, Dr. Mendelsohn explains:

"I've been asked by many companies to try their products and say nice things about them. But they were lacking in two areas: controlled studies, experimental and human, and toxicological studies. The first to demonstrate effectiveness, and the second to demonstrate safety."

"Bio-Strath has a wealth of supporting research - scientific studies carried out at the world's most prestigious medical centers and published in the world's most authoritative medical journals."

"I tried it. And to this day it remains the only food supplement I've ever taken. I believe in the Bio-Strath formula of *Candida utilis* and wild, active herbs."

"Based on the scientific studies, I support the belief that Bio-Strath can help people who experience daily tiredness, fatigue, and difficult concentration; that it may stimulate the immune system; and may actually help us assimilate more natural fuel from the foods we eat."

Lendon H. Smith, M.D. - Dr. Smith is the author of two runaway best sellers, *Foods for Healthy Kids*, and *Dr. Lendon Smith's Low Stress Diet*. In addition, he's everybody's favorite talk-show guest, lectures widely, and is a highly respected pediatrician with a large practice. This is what Dr. Lendon Smith has to say about Bio-Strath:

"Being a doctor who's also a frequent speaker, I travel a lot. When you're a doctor, people everywhere want to tell you what's bothering them. Do you know what the most common complaint is? Fatigue. And do you know what the most common cause is? The foods we eat."

"That's why I'm so excited about Bio-Strath. It contains most of the essential nutrients lost in the processing of so-called 'fast food.' This unique *Candida utilis* yeast and wild herb formula is rich in a cell energy enzyme called ATP, plus the B-vitamins, trace minerals, and other enzymes the body needs to digest and metabolize what we eat."

"These enzymes make the body work and the brain work. They're responsible for the level of energy we bring to our daily routines. And they're all in Bio-Strath. Every home should have a bottle and everyone in the family, young and old, should take a spoonful or two every day."

MIND THE DOCTORS - You won't often find two such respected and well known medical doctors speaking out in favor of an over-the-counter product. Only the scientific research and documented benefits of Bio-Strath could have convinced both Dr. Mendelsohn and Dr. Smith to lend the weight of their considerable prestige to this all-natural Swiss formula and to go public with their endorsements.

Bio-Strath is available nationwide in major health food stores and by mail order from the distributor listed in the final chapter. Along with Dr. Robert S. Mendelsohn and Dr. Lendon H. Smith, we personally recommend Bio-Strath as a quality nutritional dietary supplement, probably the finest of its kind in the world today.

The Scandinavian Dry Brush Massage

A Centuries Old Health & Beauty Secret

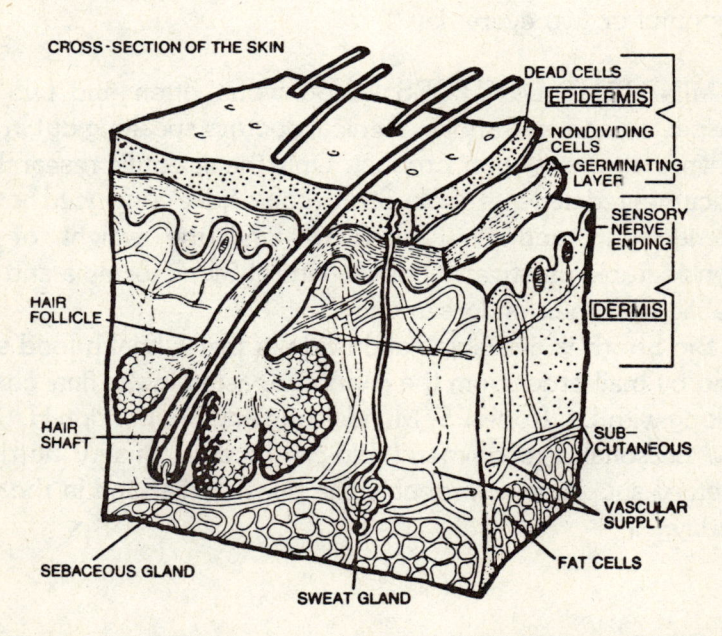

CROSS-SECTION OF THE SKIN

- DEAD CELLS
- EPIDERMIS
- NONDIVIDING CELLS
- GERMINATING LAYER
- SENSORY NERVE ENDING
- DERMIS
- HAIR FOLLICLE
- HAIR SHAFT
- SUB-CUTANEOUS
- VASCULAR SUPPLY
- SEBACEOUS GLAND
- SWEAT GLAND
- FAT CELLS

Will it surprise you to learn that the skin is the largest eliminative organ of the body? It works in a three-fold partnership with the kidneys and the liver, but the skin itself is designed to excrete as much as one pound of waste every day. When the pores of the skin are clogged with millions of dead cells, metabolic waste and toxic impurities are trapped.

CHAPTER 14

The Scandinavian Dry Brush Massage

A Centuries Old Health & Beauty Secret

The healthy, glowing skin of rosy, blond Scandinavian beauties is legendary. Do you ever wonder how they maintain that blooming luminescent luster? This all-over roseate glow stems from both a clean body and a fresh, clean constantly renewed skin. In many parts of Europe and in all the Scandinavian countries, men and women routinely practice an ages-old health and beauty technique known as the Dry Brush Massage.

The Skin Is An Important Organ

WHAT IT DOES—Although we don't think of our skin as an organ, it is - and a very important one, too. The purpose of our skin is not just to clothe the muscles and sinews that we use to move about. The skin acts as a barrier, protecting the more vulnerable interior of the body from harmful bacteria. The skin breathes, absorbing oxygen and exhaling carbon dioxide. Nutrients are absorbed through the skin. Studies have shown that the skin can assimilate certain vitamins, minerals, and proteins when they are applied topically. In the presence of sunlight, the skin produces Vitamin D which is then taken into the system through the skin.

Perhaps even more important, the skin is our largest eliminative organ and is a vital and working part of this self-cleansing miracle we call the body. As much as one-third of all impurities and toxins are excreted through the skin, exiting via hundreds and thousands of almost microscopic sweat glands. *More than one pound of metabolic waste is discharged by this incredibly complex eliminative organ every day.* In fact, chemical analysis confirms that the constituents of sweat are almost identical to that of urine.

DEFINING THE PROBLEM—The pores of the skin can become clogged with millions of dead cells, leaving it silently gasping and choking on impurities and waste it is unable to excrete. If this vital living organ slows down on its housekeeping chores, a lot of uric acid, metabolic waste, toxins, and other impurities will simply stay in the body. Of course, as a self-cleansing organism, the body will try to keep up with all the poisons and wastes that have to be eliminated daily in order for us to stay healthy.

The liver and the kidneys, our other primary waste processing organs, will attempt to compensate when the skin isn't doing its share of the job. Unfortunately, detoxifying the body is a threefold partnership. Working alone, the liver and kidneys may find themselves first overworked, then weakened, and eventually diseased. With nowhere else to go, the one pound of impurities skin is designed to excrete daily will end up as deposits in the tissues.

Because we are creatures who dearly love our comforts, we live in temperature-controlled shelters that isolate us from the elements. Thanks to modern technology, we stay effortlessly warm in winter and cool in summer. Some of us work hard and/or play hard outdoors and work up a healthy skin-stimulating sweat, but many of us labor in corporate buildings and choose sedentary indoor pleasures for our leisure activities. We never stop to realize that sweating promotes health, and that the skin needs the stimulation of changes in temperature plus fresh air to breathe in order to do its work efficiently.

Presenting The Solution

DRY BRUSH MASSAGE—The Dry Brush Massage is a health and beauty secret that brings many, many benefits. In addition, once you regularly practice this sensuous technique, either alone or with a reciprocating partner, you'll count it as one of life's greater pleasures.

Beginning with its important health benefits, here's what the Dry Brush Massage can do: (1) The millions of dry, dead cells clogging your pores will be brushed away, leaving your pores open to do their cleansing work. The capacity of your skin to excrete impurities will be immeasurably enhanced. (2) The tiny capillaries carrying blood to the surface of your skin will be energized and your entire circulatory system will be stimulated. This effect benefits all the organs and tissues of the body. (3) From the tiniest nerves in the skin throughout the entire body, the tingle will tell that your nervous system has been awakened and revitalized. (4) Keeping your skin healthy means that the impurities which lead to premature aging are excreted before they can do any damage. (5) Exercising and stimulating the millions of cells that comprise the skin will make you feel better all over and bring you a new awareness and appreciation of your healthy body.

The beauty benefits of the Dry Brush Massage offer both men and women the glow that comes from healthy well-functioning skin: (1) The appearance of your complexion will improve. As dead cells are brushed away, that dead, muddy look will disappear. (2) The hormone and oil-producing glands which moisturize the skin and keep it elastic and young-looking will be stimulated and rejuvenated. (3) You'll discover a firming and tightening effect all over your body that contributes to improved muscle tone. (4) Fat deposits of hard-to-get-rid-of cellulite will be loosened and redistributed. (5) Because signs of premature aging come from years of accumulated toxins and impurities, you'll look younger longer simply by insuring that your skin is brushed clean and able to function at optimum efficiency.

THE RIGHT BRUSH—It is very important that you understand the importance of securing a *natural bristle brush* for your Dry Brush Massage. Man-made bristles have needle-sharp ends which hurt and which can seriously damage the skin. Ideally, your brush should be made with natural pig bristles and should be equipped with a long handle so that you can reach all parts of your body. Buy one for each member of the family, please. Remember, you will actually be brushing away toxins and impurities along with a lot of dead flakes of old skin.

If you find natural bristle brushes too costly or too hard to locate, the coarse natural sponges known as *loofahs* are available in health food stores nationally and are acceptable for our purposes. Supermarkets, drug stores, and hardware stores usually stock the *plant-fiber vegetable brushes* that housewives use to scrub vegetables. If you're in a hurry to get started on your first experience with the Dry Brush Massage, a vegetable brush is very harsh, but will do.

THE DRY BRUSH MASSAGE TECHNIQUE—Start with a light touch until your body becomes used to the stimulation this technique provides. Certain parts of the body are more sensitive than others, including the face, inner-thighs, abdomen, and chest, and may require patient and gentle conditioning before they can stand real brushing.

With a clean brush — and very lightly at first — massage the skin of your face and neck in a series of gentle circles. Using the same circular motion, go next to the soles of your feet and work upward. After a thorough brushing of the feet, continue up the legs. Work the hands and arms next, followed by your chest, back, abdomen, and buttocks.

Enjoy the stimulation this technique provides and continue until your whole body is glowing, warm, and flushed rosy with healthy blood. The average time required to practice the Dry Brush Massage is between five and ten minutes. When you become used to this rejuvenating treatment, you'll find that you can use a firmer pressure with the brush. Don't hesitate to use as much firmness as you can tolerate.

As you brush, you will be amazed to find your entire body becomes coated with a fine white dust-like substance. These are the dead skin cells and impurities which have been clogging your pores. Follow your massage with a shower (or a brisk rub-down with a towel) to remove this layer of used skin.

It's a good idea to wash your brush immediately in hot water to flush away all the dead cells clinging to the bristles. Put the brush aside, bristles down, to dry thoroughly so that it's clean and pure and ready for your next massage session.

THE HOT & COLD SHOWER—The hardy folk of Scandinavia often incorporate a brisk hot and cold shower with their Dry Brush Massage. This type of shower, taken either before or after the massage, adds to the stimulating effect of the brushing. Authorities say the benefits of an alternating hot and cold shower are very real. Not only does this type of shower stimulate all the vital functions of the body, including the glandular system, it energizes the skin as well.

If you want to try the hot & cold shower before or after your Dry Brush Massage, here are a few guidelines: Stand under a very hot shower for about three minutes or until you feel heated clear through to the bone. Flip the controls to cold and splash around for about twenty seconds. Repeat the procedure three times, but always end with the water as cold as you can take it. Finish with a warming rubdown with a rough towel.

However, if the very thought of a hot and cold shower leaves you shivering in distaste, by all means take yours at the temperature you find most comfortable. All by itself, the Dry Brush

Massage technique provides the considerable and very effective stimulation the skin needs in order to act efficiently as an important eliminative organ.

THE AFTERBATH AFTERMATH - Once your whole body has been brushed glowing clean, your skin will no longer be clogged with dead cells. Flush all the impurities down the drain along with the bath water and use a natural oil to restore the skin's moisture balance. A good moisturizing oil can play an important part in maintaining and/or restoring the elasticity of youth.

For a unisex oil that will please both the most feminine and most masculine, try perfuming your blend with sandalwood. The oldest surviving written record of this naturally aromatic wood oil comes from Egypt and dates back to 1700 B.C. Sandalwood has been used for centuries as a fragrant and favored body ointment.

However, if you prefer to be pampered with a ready-made face and body-care massage oil shown in exhaustive clinical testing to eliminate fine-line wrinkles and which actually can give the entire body the taut skin of youth, the following chapter reveals a new entry in the American marketplace that actually promises these benefits! Read on...

CHAPTER 15

The Care & Feeding Of The Skin

Retarding The Natural Aging Process

After you have followed the suggestions in the previous chapter and are practicing Dry Brush Massage (see Chapter 14) on a regular basis, what's next? Once all the dead cells clogging your pores have been brushed away and your skin is breathing free and flushed with renewed health, is that all? That self-renewing miracle, the skin, is a fast healer, but it will respond visibly to further assistance, especially as we grow older.

The Age Factor

UNDER AGE TWO - From the time of birth to old age, the skin is constantly changing. Children under two years of age sweat irregularly, their sebaceous (oil secreting) glands function minimally and they have little hair. Babies and young children have clear, velvety-soft skin, unmarked by wrinkles or blemishes. The old expression, "as soft as a baby's bottom," says it all.

ADOLESCENCE - Skin pigmentation increases and *acne*, the curse of a teenager's life, very often develops. By now, hair growth (scalp, body, and the coarse facial hair of the male) is almost complete. Both the sweat glands and sebaceous secretions are functioning, sometimes profusely.

ADULT - In the young and middle-aged adult, hair growth, sweating, and sebaceous secretions have reached their full function. But continued exposures to sunlight and wind all leave indelible marks, especially on skin not protected by clothing, and a slow process of attrition commences.

OLD AGE - In the normal course of aging, the skin necessarily suffers many abuses. The moist, taut skin of youth gives way gradually to the dry, wrinkled, and flaccid skin of old age as the sebaceous glands and sweat glands slow down and function erratically.

Characteristics of the Skin

THE SURFACE—In addition to being the largest eliminative organ of the body (see Chapter 14), the skin is the largest *sensory organ* of the body as well. The millions of tiny nerves servicing the surface of the skin constantly transmit messages to the brain. The skin registers pain, responds to touch, and both monitors and regulates the exterior and internal temperature of the body constantly.

Because the skin entirely encloses and clothes the body, it plays a large part in establishing our personal identity and is therefore considered the largest organ of sexual attraction. The skin is molded, colored, and marked differently in every one of us. Each and every one of us is unique.

THE LAYERS - The skin is marvellously fashioned for maximum strength and protection from the environment, yet remains forever in communication with it. This incredible organ might be compared to plywood, which has a much greater strength than a single board of identical thickness. The skin is an array of different layers, with each possessing its own properties.

The surface of the skin (*epidermis*) is relatively thin, but is composed of four or five distinct layers. All the epidermal cells remain forever in constant and close contact with one another. But when these cells become dehydrated, the membrane at the points of adhesion between adjacent cells becomes stretched out and the skin appears dry and flakes easily.

The underlying layer (*dermis*) is somewhat thicker and is composed of two layers. One function of the dermis layer is to provide bulk for the skin. (It is interesting to note that leather is tanned dermis, with the more fragile epidermis removed and discarded.)

THE SEBACEOUS GLANDS - While the function of the sweat glands is to regulate body temperature, the *sebaceous glands* secrete *sebum*, a semiliquid mixture of fatty acids, triglycerides, waxes, cholesterol, and cellular detritus which serves as both a natural emollient and moisturizer. It is this oily secretion of the sebaceous glands which promotes elasticity and keeps the skin youthful and fresh looking.

The sebaceous glands are usually attached to hair follicles and pour their secretion into the canal of the follicle. The hairs emerging from their respective follicles and extending beyond the surface of the skin are commonly coated with a fine layer of sebum, which is transferred to the skin. The sebaceous glands are free of follicles in only a few areas of the body.

These important glands are large in newborn infants, become smaller during childhood, begin to enlarge again in early puberty, and attain full growth in adults. They are larger and more active in men than in women, and their size and efficiency of function are largely controlled by hormones.

ELASTICITY - The skin has the quite amazing ability to stretch to accommodate our changing size, either an increase (witness the tight skin of a pregnant woman's belly at full term), or a decrease (after losing a large amount of weight, for instance). Another purpose elasticity serves is to allow free movement of all body parts and muscles, from the smallest (raising one eyebrow), to the largest (kicking a football or playing golf).

Elasticity is an individual characteristic and differs widely from one person to the next. The skin of some persons is taut and resists stretching, while in others it is highly elastic and stretches easily. The degree of elasticity our skin possesses is determined by many factors, including genetics, race, and even regional differences, but is primarily age-related.

Aging is a normal part of life. Aging results from the complex interaction of physiological, psychological, and social factors. In examining the effects of aging on the skin, we find that the ability of the surface skin to adhere closely to the underlying structure, as it does in youth, is determined mainly by its elasticity. A lifetime of exposure to sun, wind, and weather certainly contributes to the characteristic wrinkles and dryness of old age, but the gradual loss of elasticity results from minimally functioning sebaceous glands and a gradual reduction in the production of the proteins *elastin* and *collagen*.

Giving Nature a Helping Hand

NOT FOR WOMEN ONLY - Not so very many years ago, it was considered decidedly less than masculine for a man to pay too much attention to his appearance. If he was clean, well-groomed, and didn't sport a 'five o'clock' shadow, he was satisfied. Only those males who made their living in the public eye (such as the stars of the theater, movies, and television) went in for facials, massages, plastic surgery, hair transplants (or hair pieces), and worked out regularly to insure that their appearance was the best it could possibly be. *Not anymore!*

Men of all ages in every walk of life all over the world are trimming down by working out. Plastic surgery is common, especially among very capable older executives who see younger men eyeing their positions with a calculating eye. Beginning years ago with the acceptable and obligatory after-shave splash, cosmetic aids for the male have now captured a large share of the market. Masculine hair sprays, gels, and even (it's about time) skin oils and moisturizers can now be found on the man's side of the bathroom medicine cabinet as well as the woman's. And that's good.

There's just no reason in this world why any of us should neglect our skin and settle for a substandard appearance when we don't have to. There are some easy techniques you can practice at home and some relatively inexpensive skin aids that will go a long way toward maintaining the firm, fresh, elastic skin of youth.

The Massage Oil

BETTER THAN A MOISTURIZER - A good massage oil is formulated specifically to encourage a massaging action, thus stimulating the surface of the skin while gently (face) or more forcefully (body) continuing the massage until the emollients are absorbed. Ideally, this type of oil should be applied to a spanking clean skin at night before retiring, and then be massaged in well. The thin sheen of oil remaining will seal in the skin's natural moisture during the night hours when the skin's natural metabolic action is enhanced.

For the best effect and almost instantly visible emprovement, enjoy a Dry Brush Massage (see Chapter 14), take a shower (or bath), and use all-over massage oil just before going to bed. An additional bonus you can expect from using this technique is the relaxation it provides, with a good night's sleep virtually assured. For pure unadulterated luxury, exchange an oil massage with a loving partner.

THE EXCEPTIONAL OIL - The absolutely best all-over massage oil we've found comes from Europe and carries impeccable U.S. credentials as well. This oil, marketed in America under the trademarked name of *frei öl* (free oil), has undergone exhaustive clinical testing by the Essex Testing Clinic, an independent testing laboratory in New Jersey. The results of these tests show that *frei öl* is totally hypoallergenic and safe for the most tender and sensitive skin.

Even more important, the final report from this prestigious institution shows that *frei öl* has almost miraculous properties. Their 1985 clinical report, entitled "Clinical Safety Evaluation of the Skin Firming & Wrinkle-Reducing (Fine Lines) Efficacy of Frei Öl," concludes with the following irrefutable statements:

"Under the conditions of an unbiased evaluation of skin firming efficacy and reduction in the incidence and depth of fine-line wrinkling, frei öl *effected an immediate (10 minute) improvement in skin firming around eye areas of the face. Following one week of daily treatment, highly significant improvements in skin firming (and increased skin elasticity) in addition to highly significant reductions in the incidence and depth of fine-line wrinkling, were observed."*

EMPIRICAL EVIDENCE - This European company has amassed a wealth of empirical evidence on the powers of *frei öl* from extremely happy users around the world. For your review, we are including a sampling of excerpts from their letters.

"Because of my husband's work, we lived in the jungles of Brazil for 30 years and I had become terribly wrinkled and dried-out from the constant sun. When we returned home, I was actually embarrassed to be seen. Despite it all, I tried *frei öl*. I was amazed to find that after only one week, I could see the difference in my skin! I will continue using this oil for the rest of my days. I was 73 when I first began using *frei öl* and I tell everyone that's it's never too late for improvement. Thank you and thank you again!" Mrs. *Eulalia O.*

"At age 15, my daughter lost 25 pounds within just a few months. Her hips and thighs were left with ugly stretchmarks, but regular massage with *frei öl* has completely eliminated them. She is now 18, very slim, and able to wear a bikini without worrying about stretchmarks. Please accept this mother's heartfelt thanks." Mrs. *Nancy C.*

"Not only for women, but also for us men, *frei öl* is excellent! I have been using it after shaving and also after my shower and I've not found anything that could improve on this terrific oil. My friends often ask me what I do to look so young at age 68. I recommend *frei öl* to them. I tell them it's economical to use and well worth the money!" *Alfred F.*

"The stretchmarks I was left with after my last pregnancy are almost gone after six months of massaging with *frei öl*. The incredible part of my story is that my youngest son is now 17 years old. My stretchmarks were also 17 years old - and I had neglected them for all those years. This product is more than amazing - it's a miracle worker!" *Mrs. Roberta L.*

"*Frei öl* is the best thing I've ever discovered for my skin! I am in my seventies, but I still attract gentlemen in their fifties and sixties. Quite something, isn't it? I'm delighted!" *Ida H.*

"My husband and I are both in our late sixties and we still massage each other regularly with *frei öl*, as we have done for the last few years. My skin has definitely improved. It feels very soft to the touch and is supple and elastic again. My husband looks younger than ever and no longer complains of feeling dry and itchy. We both enjoy our *frei öl* massage sessions and wouldn't give them up for anything!" *Mr. & Mrs. Louis H.*

There are many other small vignettes from life we could bring you, but the following little poem from *Lisabet H.* seems to sum it all up: "*Frei öl*...yes, I have to say; Now I use it every day. My same-aged friends all wag their tongue; She ain't gettin' old, she's gettin' young!"

FREI ÖL - The secret of the scientifically documented benefits of this imported oil appears to be two-fold. First, its unique formulation of rich humectants and emollients is augmented by the addition of two important nutrients known to aid the skin. *Frei öl* contains a healthy measure of both Vitamin A and Vitamin E, plus ingredients which assist absorption. Second, this clear liquid feels oily to the touch and must be massaged into the skin, the precise quality necessary to a good massage oil. *Frei öl* isn't formulated with the unnecessary additives (emulsifiers, thickeners, stabilizers, and so on) so popular with U.S. commercial cosmetic manufacturers. It is quite simply the finest basic massage oil we've found anywhere.

Yes, you may purchase *frei öl* in major health food stores around the U.S. and, *yes*, you may order *frei öl* by mail. For your convenience, we have supplied the name of the U.S. distributor in the closing chapter of this book. One more '*yes*:' We recommend *frei öl* highly for its simple purity, its ease of application, and - most importantly - because it has been proven in clinical testing to do everything it's supposed to do, and more!

CHAPTER 16

Fluoride

Decay Preventive Or A Preventable Danger?

FLUORIDE IS POISON - It is a documented fact that as little as one-tenth of an ounce of fluoride can cause death, yet all over the country, fluoride is routinely added to city water supplies as a dental caries (cavity) preventive. Statistics from the National Academy of Sciences indicate that U.S. industries pump over 100,000 tons of fluoride waste into the atmosphere every year and dump even more (an estimated 500,000 tons) into our waters. *Yes, fluoride is an industrial waste product.* And, yes, it is this same industrial waste that is used to fluoridate our drinking water.

According to the 1983 *U.S. Pharmacopeia Volumes on Drug Information*, the following clinical signs of fluoride poisoning occur with alarming frequency among people ingesting tablets containing the amount of fluoride found in just 1 to 2 pints of fluoridated water: Black stool (tar-like), bloody vomiting, diarrhea, faintness, nausea, shallow breathing, stomach pain or cramps, tremors, unusual excitement, unusual increase in saliva, watery eyes, weakness, constipation, loss of appetite, bone involvement (aches and pains), skin rash, sore (mouth, lips), stiffness, weight loss, mottling of teeth (white, brown, or black discolorations).

Documented Fluoride Poisonings

TURKEY - A town in Kizilcaoren, Turkey has been dubbed *Das Dorf der jungen Greise*, "the village where people age before their time," by the German researchers studying this phenomenon. All the inhabitants of this area suffer from premature aging. Between the ages of 30 and 40, they develop the wrinkled skin typical of the normal 60 to 70 year old; young women give birth to dead babies after pregnancies of only 4 months duration; men of 30 are impotent; all suffer from a severe weakness of the musculoskeletal structure and walking is impossible without the support of a stick. Sick livestock slaughtered for food show diseased livers.

The slow and insidious poisoning of the villagers was uncovered by a dentist who noted the typical mottling (brown discoloration) of extreme fluoride poisoning on the teeth of all children over the age of 7 and complete discoloration of teeth in teenagers. Most adults in the village had just a few affected teeth remaining. When notified of this phenomenon, the medical staff at the University Clinic of Eskisehir, Turkey conducted an intensive investigation.

Their report concluded that, on top of the reproductive difficulties and dental involvement pervading the population, "Every single inhabitant of Kizilcaoren suffers from a bone disease with symptoms including thickening of the ankles, stiffened joints, and abnormal growth of bone substance."

In neighboring Turkish villages where water is drawn from different sources, normal health prevails. But in Das Dorf der jungen Greise, water from the village well was found to contain an extremely high naturally-occurring fluoride concentration of 5.4 ppm (parts per million).

MASSIVE U.S. FLUORIDE POISONINGS - At least the water in that Turkish well was naturally fluoridated, not knowingly poisoned by Turkish officials. But if you live in a city with artificially fluoridated water, and most of us do, you are at the mercy of a possible malfunction of the automatic equipment dispensing this poison into the water that comes into our homes. It's happened more than once.

In Annapolis, Maryland (November 1979), up to 50 ppm fluoride was accidentally pumped into the public water supply. (*This is ten times the amount documented as causing all the damage in Turkey.*) An estimated 10,000 Marylanders exhibited acute symptoms of fluoride poisoning and some 50,000 people ingested poisonous concentrations of this deadly substance. Over five times as many people died of heart attacks during the week following the malfunction than could be expected in the normal course of events. The people were not warned of the spill because, in the words of an Annapolis public health official, "We did not want to jeopardize the fluoridation program."

Other fluoride spills have occurred around the country as well. It is entirely likely that malfunctioning equipment dumps dangerous amounts of fluoride into public water supplies without our every being aware of it. Documented instances of massive fluoride spills have been found in North Carolina, Pennsylvania, California, New Mexico, Maine, Michigan, and elsewhere. State, county, and city officials go out of their way to hush up the problem.

AUSTRALIA - The death certificate of 18-month old Jason B. listed his cause of death as fluoride poisoning. Jason's mother, Mrs. B., explains: "I took fluoride tablets during my pregnancy on the advice of my doctor and Jason had been taking fluoride tablets regularly since his first birthday. Then I found Jason sitting on the floor with an open bottle of fluoride tablets. The doctor told me to take Jason to the hospital (Mater Children's Hospital, Brisbane) immediately to have his stomach pumped, which I did." (The pump disgorged four fluoride tablets from Jason's tiny stomach.)

Mrs. B. continues, "At home later, Jason became unconscious and I rushed him back to the hospital. They put a tube down his throat and hooked him up to a respirator. But four days later, a brain specialist told me that Jason was brain-dead. At first the doctors told me that it was impossible for fluoride to kill my son, but they finally admitted it was the fluoride."

A spokeman for the Queensland Justice Department has confirmed that Jason's death was caused by fluoride poisoning and that the death certificate is authentic.

UNITED STATES - Three year old William K. was the victim of fluoride poisoning when a stannous fluoride gel was applied directly to his teeth as a decay preventive. After a dental hygientist swabbed his teeth with the fluoride gel, she handed the youngster a cup of water without instructing him to rinse and spit. William drank the water and took in triple the amount of fluoride necessary to cause death.

Seeing her son immediately begin vomiting and sweating, Mrs. K. rushed him to a pediatrician in the same building. When William was examined, he was found to be in a comatose state. The pediatrician injected adrenalin into his heart to revive him and William was transported by ambulance to a nearby hospital, but he again lapsed into a coma. The doctors were attempting to pump his stomach when he went into cardiac arrest and died.

In yet another tragic case, a U.S. dental hygienist reports witnessing the almost immediate death of a child after fluoride treatment. Terry L. says, "One of my bosses was working on a patient and applied topical fluoride. The child went into convulsions and died in the chair. It happened so fast that nobody could do anything for him. It was just a few minutes after the fluoride was applied. The parents never got the true answer."

The dental clinic has refused any responsibility for the child's death. Even though there was no history of any heart problem, the clinic maintains that the child died of a heart attack.

An incident of fluoride poisoning that had a happy ending involved a five-year old participating in a program of weekly fluoride rinses at his Head Start facility. After just a month on the fluoride program, Eric M., normally a healthy active boy, developed into a sickly child. He complained of stomach aches, lost his appetite and wanted to sleep all the time. Mrs. M. was worried and took Eric to see his pediatrician. The doctor said it was just a nervous condition, but Mrs. M. rejected that explanation.

Fortunately, Mrs. M. heard of the dangers of fluoride in time to take Eric out of the fluoride rinse program. She remembers talking with an authority (Andrew Craig) and says he told her that "Fluorride is a poison and can cause gastrointestinal tract problems, especially in small children." After reading the information he gave me, I took Eric out of the program, threw away our fluoridated toothpaste, and dumped out all the fluoridated food and drinks we had in the house.

"Eric's health was 100% better after just one week of being off the fluoride. I look back now and realize how sick Eric really was. I don't want to think about what could have happened to him if we hadn't caught the fluoride poisoning in time."

Not An Acceptable Risk

DOES FLUORIDE PREVENT CAVITIES? - No. Early studies published by the U.S. Public Health Service are interpreted (by fluoride advocates) to show that children consuming water containing 1.5 ppm (parts per million) fluoride have less tooth decay than children drinking water with relatively small amounts of fluoride. *But later studies by the same agency of the federal government show no difference in tooth decay rates between high and low fluoride areas.* The cavity preventive effects originally attributed to fluoridated water have since been shown to be caused by other minerals.

You need to be aware that biased interests can easily manipulate any type of study to influence the results. For instance, the Grand Rapids-Muskegon (Michigan) study of fluoride is often cited in support of fluoridation. Here's what happened. Five years into what was supposed to be a ten-year study, fluoride advocates found that the tooth decay rate of Muskegon (nonfluoridated) had actually decreased at the same rate as that of Grand Rapids (artificially fluoridated).

Because this data did not support fluoridation, nonfluoridated

Muskegon was dropped from the study as the control city. The published report states only that the rate of tooth decay in Grand Rapids decreased during the period of the study. The inference is that artificially fluoridating the water was the cause of the drop in the rate of tooth decay. However, it has been determined conclusively that life-long residents of Grand Rapids have a tooth decay rate equal to the national average.

Japanese, British, and Danish studies mounted to evaluate the benefits of fluoride against dental caries have uniformly determined that there is no fluoride-related reduction in tooth decay rates. In fact, Japanese researchers discovered a higher percentage of students with tooth decay in areas where the fluoride levels were 0.5 ppm or more than in areas with a 0.2 to 0.4 ppm. The Japanese study comprised a group of over 20,000 students.

World-wide research shows that fluoridation of water does not influence the rate of tooth decay and is not effective in reducing these rates. The U.S. has one of the highest rates of dental caries in the world, yet is one of the most fluoridated countries in the world. The bottom line is that Americans greedily consume a diet high in refined carbohydrates, thus promoting tooth decay. In many so-called primitive societies where processed sweets are unavailable, 80 to 90 percent of the population live out their lives without tooth decay and go to the grave with a full set of perfect teeth, in spite of the fact that their drinking water contains a negligible amount of fluoride.

The Cancer Connection

THE IMMUNE SYSTEM - Scientists at the Seibersdorf Research Center in Austria have reported that as little as 1 ppm fluoride slows down the vitally important DNA repair enzyme activity of the immune system. It has long been noted that the higher incidence of cancer among older persons is directly related to the proven decline in the ability of the immune system to repair defective DNA components

Numerous laboratory studies have shown that fluoridated water (at concentrations as low as 1 ppm) can cause serious genetic and chromosomal damage in plants, animals, and humans. Using bone marrow and testes cells, a U.S. geneticist has demonstrated that the degree of chromosomal damage increases proportionately as the fluoride content of the water increases. It is important to note that abnormal sperm cells which have been damaged by fluoride poisoning can lead to serious birth defects and certain metabolic disorders that can be passed on from generation to generation.

Using the same level of fluoride commonly put into U.S. water supplies, scientists at the Nippon Dental College in Japan have determined that this minute amount of fluoride is capable of transforming normal cells into cancer cells. At a meeting of the Japanese Association of Cancer Research in Osaka in 1982, the researchers reported, "Last year at this meeting we showed that sodium fluoride, which is being used for the prevention of dental caries, induces chromosomal aberrations and irregular synthesis of DNA. This year, we report our finding that a malignant transformation of cells is induced by sodium fluoride."

As incredible as it may seem, research sponsored by the American Cancer Institute as long ago as 1963 clearly showed that even very low levels of fluoride increased the incidence of melanodic tumors in experimental laboratory animals by a frightening 12 to 100 percent. Similar types of transformations of normal cells to potentially cancerous cells have been observed in humans.

Polish scientists working at the Pomeranian Medical Academy have published reports that as little as 0.6 ppm fluoride produces chromosomal damage in human white blood cells, the important defensive cells of the immune system.

Fluoridated Communities

DRINK AT YOUR PERIL - If you walk into a store and purchase

sodium fluoride (McKesson), you will find the label carries the universal warning symbol of a Skull & Crossbones along with the words: *Warning - Poison.*

Dean Burk, Chief Chemist Emeritus of the U.S. National Cancer Institute has been quoted as saying, *"In point of fact, fluoride causes more human cancer death, and causes it faster, than any other chemical."* More than a decade ago, Dr. Dean Burk and John Yiamouyiannis Ph.D. mounted a series of studies to determine if a link between cancer and fluoridated communities could be proven. You should know that Dr. Yiamouyiannis is recognized internationally as the world's leading authority on the biological effects of fluoride. His book, *Fluoride - The Aging Factor*, published in 1983 by Health Action Press, is a dramatic expose of the dangers of fluoridation and fluoride contamination. Dr. Yiamouyiannis currently serves as president of the Safe Water Foundation with headquarters in Columbus, Ohio.

Using cities with comparable cancer death rate statistics from the ten-year period between 1940 and 1950 before fluoridation began as their control, the two scientists then selected the ten largest fluoridated cities and ten largest nonfluoridated cities and began a cross comparison. What they found was conclusive data showing a definite relationship between fluoridated water and cancer statistics.

In the period from 1952 to 1956 when fluoride was added to the water supplies of the test cities, the cancer death rate rose dramatically in comparison to the nonfluoridated cities. By 1969, the average cancer death rate in the fluoridated cities averaged between 220 and 225 cancer deaths per 100,000 people, a cancer death rate increase of approximately 10 percent in just 13 to 17 years.

ADDITIONAL FINDINGS - An even more extensive study conducted by the U.S. Center for Disease Control has confirmed an increased cancer death rate, particularly among persons 45 years and older, living in communities supplying fluoridated water. Another U.S. Public Health Service study has found a 22 percent increase in the cancer death rate in Grand Rapids, Michigan following fluoridation, in direct contrast to the nonfluoridated control city of Muskegon. The California Tumor Registry has confirmed their findings that people living in fluoridated California cities suffer a cancer death rate up to 40 percent higher than those living in non-fluoridated areas. A recent Canadian study shows 15 to 25 percent more cancer deaths in fluoridated provinces.

NEEDLESS DEATHS - According to data (corrected for age, sex, and race) supplied by the U.S. Center for Disease Control, deaths from all causes are at least 5 percent higher in areas supplying fluoridated water in comparison with nonfluoridated controls.

As if we don't have enough outside contamination to worry about, what this means is that we are deliberately drinking a known poison and carcinogen and we are infecting our children with fluoride dental treatments and urging them to brush with fluoride toothpaste.

Including the 10,000 to 20,000 deaths each year believed to be due to fluoride-induced cancer, the total number of fluoride-related deaths is estimated to be between 30,000 to 50,000. *Warning:* This figure is escalating yearly. Worst of all, we're doing it on purpose simply because we've been brainwashed into believing the mistaken notion that fluoride can reduce dental decay.

Escaping Fluoride Poisonings

WATER CONTAMINATION — If you live in a fluoridated city, we urge you to alert your loved ones, friends, and neighbors to the dangers of fluoride. Talk to city officials and let them know they've been misinformed on the benefits of fluoride. No one is knowingly going to poison the water supply and we have to believe that they honestly don't know what they're doing by dumping fluoride into city water.

In fluoridated areas, by far the largest amount of fluoride you are ingesting is from your drinking water. Consider, this water is used to dilute the baby's formula, mix up fruit juice and soft drinks, to cook soups, cereals, vegetables, to brew coffee and tea, even to make homemade bread. For your health's sake, don't drink fluoridated water or cook with it. Would you purchase a chemical carrying the Skull & Crossbones label and feed it to your family deliberately?

For unpoisoned water, use a home water distiller, have it delivered by a local supplier, or purchase steam distilled water by the jug at your local supermarket.

PURCHASED BEVERAGES & FOODS - Reconstituted fruit juices and soft drinks are usually made with fluoridated water, as are many beers and wines. The only way to find out for sure if these beverages contain fluoride is to note the area where they are bottled. The U.S. Center for Disease Control, Atlanta, Georgia 30330 will mail you a copy of a list of localities using fluoridated water. If your favorite beverage is bottled in a fluoridated area, it contains fluoride.

Tracking down fluoridated foods is a little more difficult. Any canned or otherwise packaged product which lists *water* as a major ingredient (one of the first three on the ingredient panel) may also pose a hazard. Again, determine the city of manufacture and check your list of fluoridated areas.

COMMON PRODUCTS - Discard fluoridated toothpastes, mouthwashes, vitamin tablets and vitamin drops. (Fluoride is *not* an essential nutrient and don't let anyone tell you otherwise.) Replace these common household products with nonfluoridated versions. If your supermarket doesn't have them, your local health food store will.

OTHER DANGERS - Tell your dentist politely that you don't wish your child to have fluoride applied topically to his teeth. And, for heaven's sake, tell him why! You may save someone else's child from death by fluoride poisoning. If a fluoride rinse program is operating in your neighborhood, alert the director of the program immediately to the dangers of exposing children to this poison.

Sodium fluoride is sold as an insecticide and is used as a bug and rodent killer in many schools, including the cafeteria area. There is a real danger of food contamination and the possibility of inhaling the fluoride powder. A phone call *now* to find out if your child's school is using fluoride may avoid fluoride poisoning later.

Spread the Word

SCREAM & HOLLER - Although the temptation to indulge in a little vigilante justice might be strong, forget it. Go to your community newspaper, get up a petition (not a posse), become involved in town meetings, talk to school officials (including nursery schools and Head Start facilities), and generally do your part to spread the word about the scientifically documented dangers of fluoridated water.

To protect their jobs, politicians have to listen to the voice of their consituents. If enough of us scream and holler, we can get this killer taken out of our water supplies. *You can make a difference.*

EDITORS NOTE - The material in this chapter is a prepublication release and has been excerpted from a new in-depth book on cancer entitled *How To Fight Cancer & Win* (Fisher Publishing Company, Canfield, Ohio 44406), still in manuscript form. The author agreed that this information could be of such vital importance to the American public that it should be made available immediately and not held pending future publication.

CHAPTER 17

Little-Known Cancer Preventives & Some Avoidable Carcinogens

Controversial Findings From Around the World

HOW GOES THE WAR? - Since 1971 when former President Richard Nixon decreed an all-out war on cancer, we have spent over 20 billion dollars in an attempt to discover a cure for this most feared disease. How are we doing? Trying to keep score is difficult.

In 1962, 170 persons in every 100,000 died of cancer. In 1982, the tally was 185 persons in every 100,000. On the surface, it appears that the incidence of cancer has gone up an alarming 9 percent in the last twenty years. But the American Cancer Society points out that it is the escalation of lung cancer rates (tied inescapably to a proportionate escalation in smoking) which has caused the increase. The ACS points out that the death rate for most other cancers remains approximately the same as it was in 1962. According to ACS projections, over one million Americans will be diagnosed as having some form of cancer in 1986.

Is that good enough? Dr. John C. Bailar doesn't think we've received sufficient value for our money. The well respected *New England Journal of Medicine* (May 1986) carried an article authored by John C. Bailar, M.D. of the School of Public Health at Harvard. Dr Bailar contends that we are losing the war against cancer and puts forth a recommendation that he believes will go a long way toward solving the problem.

Dr. Bailar has come out four-square in favor of a preventive approach to the cancer dilemma. Rather than spending our total funds trying to find a cancer cure-all, in effect trying to close the barn door after the horse has been stolen, Dr. Bailar suggests that researchers concentrate instead on discovering ways to prevent the disease from occurring in the first place. He suggests that for every dollar spent on researching a cure, two dollars be spent on researching preventive measures. We agree. A preventive approach will certainly benefit all of us now living and may eliminate the spectre of cancer hanging heavy over the heads of future generations as well. ·

Researchers around the world have been coming up with some startling data, much of which is ignored by our U.S. scientists. Although most of the findings from various parts of the globe regarding cancer preventives and/or cancer therapies are based on sound scientific theory and are founded on impressive clinical research, very little of this vital information has been made available to the American public until now.

However, as more and more irrefutable data is published, it is expected that public demand will force the U.S. to sit up and take notice. For instance, certain compounds in widespread use in the European theatre and many other parts of the world, including the United States, have been termed "quackery" by the orthodox medical community of the U.S. and are therefore unavailable in this country. Even some vitally important U.S. findings have been suppressed and the tests distorted.

Laetrile - A Case in Point

The name *Laetrile*, an apricot pit formula which was developed at the John Beard Memorial Foundation in San Francisco, is a registered trademark coined in 1952 by its discoverer, Ernst Krebs, Jr. Laetrile is a combination of the term *laevorotary* (having the ability to turn polarized light to the left) and *nitrile* (an organic compound in which nitrogen exists with all three of the displaced hydrogen atoms). Just as the registered trademark 'Kleenex' has come to mean any kind of nose-tissue, so Laetrile is commonly misused as a generic term for *amygdalin* (B-17)

AMYGDALIN - Amygdalin is found in over a thousand foods, one or more of which most of us eat every day. Lettuce, corn, kidney beans, sugar cane, millet, cassava, sorghum, lima beans, sweet potatoes and linseed all contain amygdalin. Strawberries, raspberries, blackberries, boysenberries, cranberries, elderberries, mulberries, gooseberries, huckleberries, loganberries and chokeberries furnish amygdalin. (Note: Amygdalin is more abundant in wild berries than in cultivated.) And, although we don't usually crunch the hard pits of the following popular fruits, amygdalin is also present in the seeds of apples, apricots, bitter almonds, cherries, peaches, plums, and prunes. (Note: Our sweet almonds contain very little amygalin. Bitter almonds, an important part of Chinese medicine, are not available in the U.S.)

Amygdalin contains a natural cyanide compound which is not toxic in the human body and this natural form of cyanide is of immense value in cancer treatment. The malignant cell contains a special enzyme which releases the poison in amygdalin. The poison, in turn, attacks the malignant cell and assists in its destruction. Normal cells do not contain this special enzyme, do not release the cyanide, and therefore remain unchanged and unharmed.

When a correlation of data provides a comparison of people who ingest foods high in amygdalin versus those who do not, we may find an important clue to why some individuals contract cancer while others do not. If we are continually providing our body with foods containing amygdalin, known to attack and destroy cancer cells, how then can a malignancy grow and spread? Amygdalin will almost certainly prove to be an exceptionally efficient cancer-preventive.

The difference between amygdalin and Laetrile is that Laetrile contains amygdalin changed by a patented process from a glucoside to glucuronic acid. When amygdalin itself is ingested, either in foods or as an extracted compound, the conversion process from glucose to glucuronic acid takes place in the liver. Because Laetrile is already a glucuronic acid, the body does not have to initiate the conversion process. (Note: Extracted amygdalin is highly unstable in liquid form. Only dry, crystallized amygdalin is considered therapeutically active.)

Even though bitter almonds, probably the most abundant source of natural amygdalin, have been used in Chinese herbal medicine since 2800 B.C., the F.D.A. (U.S. Food & Drug Administration) does not consider the natural compound Laetrile a food, but has instead termed it a "drug." As the champion and sponsor of Laetrile, the McNaughton Foundation has handled all the red-tape and paper work necessary to bring this compound to the world.

By the end of 1978, more than 20 states had ruled that their citizens had a right to choose Laetrile as a holistic and nontoxic treatment for cancer and all seemed well. But approximately a year later, the National Cancer Institute filed an I.N.D. (Investigational New Drug) application and Phase II testing of Laetrile was scheduled. It is important to note that a Phase II test is allowed *only* after Phase I testing proves that the material being tested is not toxic in prescribed amounts.

What happened in the Phase II testing to give Laetrile such bad publicity? First and foremost, whether by accident or design, *the material the NCI tested was not therapeutically-active natural Laetrile-amygdalin.*

According to Laetrile supporters, there were other serious problems with the test as well. For instance, only terminal cancer patients were selected for the study, patients whose immune systems had already been completely destroyed, either by the disease or by the orthodox medical treatments which had been administered prior to the test. And, although the documented side-effects of chemotherapy and radiation therapy (permitted by the F.D.A.) are certainly toxic and also destroy normal cells and tissue, any patient in the so-called Laetrile study who complained of something as slight as a mild headache was immediately taken out of the program and chalked up on the negative side of the ledger.

Some Laetrile advocates say there were other built-in negatives in the study as well and infer that the test was programmed so carefully that Laetrile was bound to fail. At a meeting of the Society of Clinical Oncology on April 30, 1981, Charles Moertel, M.D., of the prestigious Mayo Clinic announced, "Laetrile has been tested. It is not effective."

THE FIGHT GOES ON - Not only for laetrile-amygdalin, but for the basic right of the American public to choose the type of health care they want for themselves. Alternative nutritional and holistic therapies of all kinds are under attack. If you want to join the battle or want more detailed information, contact The National Health Federation, Monrovia, California 91016.

The bureaucratic management of the Laetrile affair makes a very clear point. If a *U.S.* researched and developed non-toxic nutritional cancer therapy of proven value can't make it through the system, what chance is there that cancer preventives, treatments, and/or therapies used with such success in other parts of the world will ever be made available to the American public?

And what about known carcinogens and poisons that are not only permitted to infiltrate the food chain (in approved fertilizers) and the water supplies of U.S. cities? Some, like fluoride, are actually promoted as being good for us. See *Fluoride* (Chapter 16).

Dateline Europe

GERMANY - One of the most comprehensive treatises on disease prevention and cure currently in publication is a scholarly work by the world famous Hans Nieper, M.D. entitled *Revolution in Technology, Medicine & Society.* Although this important book has been published in English as well as German, you won't find it in many local bookstores or even your neighborhood library. This work delves deeply into the causes of all the common diseases of civilization, including cancer, and explains some of the most successful methods of both treatment and prevention.

GENE-REPAIRING TREATMENT - Dr. Nieper says, "Some of the gene-repairing therapeutic measures for cancer, as well as protective measures for cancer, are already available and others will be added. Therapy should be applied immediately after the first discovery of, or operation on, a malignant tumor. This is mandatory. Any waiting game is fundamentally wrong. Modern gene-repairing therapy is practically nontoxic. It represents, so to speak, an imitation of the cancer defense of our body. Today there is no longer any doubt about its highly clinical value." In this chapter, we will briefly detail the findings, preventives, and treatments discussed in this serious work, plus outline the factors which are known to add to the risk of contracting cancer.

Dietary Considerations

THE FOOD FACTOR - As a very graphic example of the chemical changes certain foods exert within the body, consider the case of a respected German physician which was presented at the Baden-Baden cancer congress last year. This physician used himself as an experimental tool to prove a point. After eating a meal of fried chicken, the doctor demonstrated that the malignant tumor in his neck was well-nourished and grew rapidly. In direct contrast, he found that a whole-grain diet of millet caused the tumor to be drastically reduced. In fact, the millet diet proved more effective in shrinking the tumor than orthodox chemotherapy.

This case alone proves that the body is influenced daily by nutrient intake. Diet plays a vital part in the day-to-day functioning of the body and does not merely affect the body over the long-term, as most authorities believe.

According to Dr. Nieper, the dietary recommendations of the U.S. Department of Health, Education and Welfare for a cancer-protective diet are incomplete in that there is no mention of the importance of Vitamins C and D2, magnesium, molybdenum, selenium, and beta-carotene in reducing the risk of contracting cancer.

OBESITY - Another factor which is stressed by knowledgeable oncologists is the importance of *under-eating*. Unfortunately, Americans in particular commonly overeat. While an occasional holiday feast will not increase the long-term risk of developing cancer (as long as only the proper foods are enjoyed), carrying even a mere ten pounds over your ideal weight can add to your risk. A U.S. study conducted by Bayer Pharmaceuticals clearly showed that the incidence of cancer was reduced in laboratory mice especially bred to develop mammary cancer when they were consistently underfed. The healthiest exercise in the world still remains pushing yourself away from the table after a meager meal. Clearly, gluttony is one of the deadliest of the seven deadly sins.

Although German health authorities have not publicized a cancer-preventive diet, the recommendations contained in Dr. Nieper's book, *Revolution in Technology, Medicine & Society*, follow. It is interesting to note that these recommendations are very similar to the recommendations of the U.S. National Research Council.

PREFERRED FOODS - *(1)* Whole grain breads, oatmeal, millet, *(2)* skim milk, *(3)* fish (in limited quantity), *(4)* fruit and fiber-rich vegetables (cooked and raw), *(5)* carrot juice, *(6)* pancreatic enzyme supplements, *(7) Omniflora** capsules, *Eupalan** bifidum flora containing milk. (*German preparations)

RESTRICTED FOODS - *(1)* No meat; no sausage, (6 or 7 ounces meat per week is permitted in cases of exhaustion, lack of blood protein, or cachexia), *(2)* little cheese, *(3)* very little sugar, *(4)* very little fast-release carbohydrates (pastries, puddings, manufactured sweets), *(5) no shellfish* (because of its high nuclein content), *(6)* no smoking, *(7)* no 'junk' beverages (carbonated sodas, etc.), *(8)* no apple juice (too high in glucose), *(9)* no distilled water.

Some of the most important anti-cancer nutrients targeted in this serious work follow, along with an explanation of the work they perform within the body.

BETA-CAROTENE - This important element is a *precursor* of Vitamin A. In other words, the body uses beta-carotene to manufacture Vitamin A. Unlike Vitamin A, research has shown that beta-carotene does not harm the liver. With their rich content of beta-carotene, carrots are considered an excellent natural preventive. For the full story on beta-carotene, please see *Carrots* (Chapter 2).

Note: Chapter 4 also discusses over-the-counter beta-carotene preparations available through some health food stores. If you don't find it convenient to include carrots in your daily diet, please review Chapter 4 before purchasing beta-carotene in prepared form.

SELENIUM - Selenium is an important element currently under investigation around the world as a possible aid to a healthy heart. Many heart patients who have fallen victim to a cardiac arrest or cardiac infarction have been shown to be deficient in selenium. Respected authorities believe selenium affords strong protection against cancer as well.

However, it has become difficult to take in enough selenium in the average diet. Soil studies show that many food-producing areas of the world lack selenium in their growing fields. If the nutrient is not available in the soil, it cannot be present in the food. A selenium deficiency is very common among the populations of the civilized world.

MAGNESIUM - A 10-year long German study has shown that patients taking magnesium (aspartate and orotate) therapy for heart disease have a 20 percent less incidence of cancer than occurs in the normal population mix. This research validates the observation that in regions where the drinking water is high in magnesium, there is a much lower rate of both cancer and heart disease.

Magnesium is known to enrich the body's immune defense system by assisting in the production of antibodies and strengthening the white blood cells. Magnesium is helpful to many other functions which maintain normal cell development as well. Since a malignancy is caused by abnormal cell development, it's easy to see why magnesium is a necessary cancer preventive.

A diet which includes a lot of whole-grains, fruits, and vegetables should supply sufficient magnesium for healthy functioning. Authorities say that a dangerously low level of magnesium is rare, but can occur. For instance, a junk-food diet, chronic diarrhea, or a condition which interferes with proper assimilation of nutrients can set the stage for a magnesium deficiency.

SODIUM - Although sodium is rarely found in the makeup of a normal cell, the abnormal cancerous cell pumps sodium into itself. When a cell goes haywire and becomes malignant, it loses the calcium lining of its inner membranes, with magnesium and potassium also being lost. With the loss of calcium, the cell loses its normal defense capabilities. By absorbing sodium, the cancer cell places itself beyond the body's normal defenses.

The blood analyses of cancer patients commonly show that not only the malignancy, but the blood cells themselves are overloaded with sodium. A promising theory suggests that removing the sodium (desodification) from the cancer cells would open them once more to the body's immune system defenses. But what substance can modern medicine offer to selectively remove the sodium from the cancer cells? The answer to this problem may yet come from a killer who lives in the depths of the oceans.

Currently in Research

SQUALENE - In the human body and in all animals, cancer rarely finds a home in the cartilage. But the cartilage of the shark's fin is even more resistant to cancer than human cartilage. In fact, as a species, sharks appear to have a built-in protection against cancer, and not just in their fin cartilage either. A study conducted under the auspices of the Smithsonian Institute in Washington, D.C. discovered only one malignant tumor in 25,000 sharks!

The shark secretes certain substances (taurine and isaethionic acid) in its liver which constantly recycle the high salt concentration of its environment back into the sea. In current medical practice, taurine is often prescribed for both migraine headaches and epilepsy. The shark's anticancer potential is incredibly high because it is in a constant process of desodification.

The shark has yet another method of suppressing cancer. Along with its ability to eliminate sodium, the shark produces an oily substance called squalene. Squalene is produced in large quantities in the shark's liver and is also found in smaller amounts in both cod liver oil and olive oil. Researchers believe that squalene restores the vital electrostatic balance which is lost when a cell turns cancerous. Once the balance is restored by the squalene, the body's defense system can identify, attack, and destroy the malignancy.

DHEA - DHEA (dehydroepiandrosterone) levels in the blood apparently play a protective role against the development of cancer. It has been determined that when DHEA levels in the blood rise to a value of more than 3.3 mg, a cancer tumor goes into remission. Squalene appears to stimulate the body's own production of DHEA. It is known that approximately 60 percent of the population contains sufficient natural DHEA to be protected from cancer. Of the remaining 40 percent deficient in DHEA, it is theorized that more than half (22 percent) will die from cancer.

ALDEHYDES - The 'bitter almond' (Mandelonitrile) substances exert a gene-repairing effect on cancer cells. These substances include amygdalin, prunasin, cassavin, ficin, and the synthetic mandelonitril compounds. Benzaldehyde (one of the constituents of Laetrile) has been shown to have a very positive effect against cancer cells. The excellent experimental and clinical results achieved in Japan with benzaldehyde treatments were published by the National Cancer Institute as long ago as 1980.

Various forms of aldehyde cancer therapy have been practiced in Germany at the Paracelsus Hospital in Hannover for more than 15 years. A respected head nurse with many years of experience working with cancer patients at this prestigious institution says without hesitation, "Among all forms of medical cancer treatment, including poisonous chemotherapy, this is still the best method."

RUBIDIUM & CESIUM - Both are nontoxic elements shown to be absorbed by a cancer cell. Once absorbed, they neutralize the harmful hydrogen ions present in the malignancy. Studies indicate that this treatment has a positive effect even when a cancer growth has attained considerable volume, but primarily assists the body's own immune system. These elements should therefore be administered early, before the defenses of the body have been damaged beyond repair.

UREA - Urea is a natural product of metabolized protein long used in medicine as a diuretic and in the diagnosis of kidney function. Urea therapy is considered inexpensive, harmless, and can be used for a long period. Results achieved at the Greek Cancer Clinic as far back as the early 1970's show that urea has strong antiviral properties and is therefore effective against viral-induced malignancies, such as liver cancer (hepatitis B) and oral tumors (herpes virus).

As a powerful diuretic, urea has been shown to detoxify the body by eliminating cancer degradation byproducts. The Greek studies published in 1974 list several case histories of cancer patients then in remission after receiving between 10 and 18 grams of urea daily.

Assisting Internal Defense Mechanisms

STEROIDS - Certain lymphocytes (white blood cells) play a very important part in the defense systems of the body. Lymph cells function efficiently only when they are present in sufficient quantity. In order to possess the ability to inactivate a cancerous cell, lymphocytes require special steroids: *thymosterine* and *tumosterone*. In order to manufacture tumosterone, the body must first manufacture its precursor, thymosterine. And, in order to be able to manufacture the precursor thymosterine, the body requires Vitamin D2. Prednisone (but no other cortisone) is also a precursor of thymosterine. The steroids thymosterine and tumosterone are both activated by the thymus gland. A healthy thymus gland is absolutely vital to an efficiently functioning immune system.

It is believed that tumosterone moves directly into the nucleus of the malignant cell via the lymph and inactivates it. However, this can only occur if a lymphocyte with sufficient tumosterone has identified and attached itself to the cancer cell.

German researchers have broken down tumosterone chemically and have succeeded in identifying the final metabolite of this protective element as 7-beta-hydroxycholsterol. This means that tumosterone can now be produced in a laboratory.

SHEEP LICE - Sheep are extremely resistant to cancer, possibly because their wool-fat has been shown to be especially rich in tumosterone. An old-country cure for viral hepatitis has been practiced in Germany for centuries. It consists of eating sheep lice. This is just one more demonstration of a folk medicine strongly rooted in what we now know to be scientific fact.

Although it is difficult to stimulate the functioning of the thymus gland directly, science can provide elements which assist the immune system. A continuing intake of bromelaine, abundant in pineapples, may be a useful aid to the immune system and is considered an excellent cancer-preventive as well. Gamma-globulin, zinc-aspartate, manganese-aspartate, and molybdenum (abundant in cauliflower), are considered helpful. It has been noted that zinc enhances the body's defenses against cancer and exerts a pronounced preventive effect. But, caution must be observed. Once a malignant tumor has become established, zinc may increase its rate of growth.

ANTITUBERCULOSIS VACCINE - Over twenty years ago, researchers discovered that an injection of the antituberculosis vaccine BCG (Calmette-Guerin bacillus) can activate two or three different defense procedures of the white blood corpuscles. Clinical trials showed that these internal defenses can be dramatically effective, even against advanced cancer. The use of the vaccine demands particular care, however. Unless the body's immune system is still functioning, the vaccine may shut it down entirely.

At Increased Risk

Certain whole segments of the population are, on average, at increased risk of developing some type of cancer within their lifetimes. For instance, employment in the rayon industry carries a higher cancer risk, just as miners risk developing black lung. Predicting who will and who will not develop a malignancy within any given group of persons is not an exact science because so many diverse factors influence health.

However, the following information deserves your close attention. You just might find that you or someone you love is in a high-risk group without even being aware of it. Identifying high-risk groups is the first step to assisting these groups in lowering their risk. This very vital information is unknown to most of the American public.

BLOOD TYPE A - Cancer cells develop a defense mechanism

of their own by surrounding themselves with a camouflaging layer of mucus. This protective outer layer makes it difficult for the body's own defenses to recognize a malignant cell and they hesitate to attack it.

Those of us with blood type A are at particular risk of developing cancer at some time in our lives because cancerous cells have a marked resemblance to blood type A cells. The defense system present in blood group A is not efficient in identifying cancer cells and is very slow to attack, thereby giving the cancer a better chance of developing.

German research has documented this problem. Blood type A represents 43 percent, less than half, of the German population. But a whopping 77 percent, more than three-quarters, of the cancer victims in that nation are blood type A. At the opposite end of the scale, the study showed that only 19 percent of Germany's cancer patients are blood type O, but blood type O carriers represents the highest percentage of the general population.

Clearly, blood type A (AB) carriers should incorporate all the preventive measures known into their lifestyles as quickly as possible in order to reduce their high risk of developing cancer.

THE FAMILY AT RISK - It has long been noted that being born into a cancer-prone family appears to increase your risk of developing a malignancy at some time in your life. The American Institute for Cancer Research has begun an all-out offensive to discover why cancer seems to run in certain families.

The research has zeroed in on one particular oncogene called the Ha-*ras* gene. The term *oncogene* comes from the Greek word 'oncos' or tumor. Scientists theorize that oncogenes are present in all cells and believe their function is to regulate cell growth. Because cancer cells grow abnormally, learning what factor regulates normal cell growth is vitally important. Once the growth factor is identified, medical science may be able to develop a procedure to control the abnormal proliferation of cancer cells.

When viewed under a powerful electronic microscope, the Ha-

ras gene reveals as many as 20 distinct different patterns. In an intensive study of this particular oncogene, both cancer patients and those in the control group were shown to carry four of the most common patterns. Of the sixteen less common Ha-*ras* patterns, 12 were found only in cancer patients.

This important research indicates that persons carrying the Ha-*ras* gene in one of the 12 suspect configurations are at higher risk of contracting cancer than their brothers and sisters who may not have inherited one of the problem patterns. Science may soon be able to perform a simple blood test to determine your genetic risk of developing a malignancy.

If you carry one of the Ha-*ras* genes commonly found in cancer patients, it does not automatically follow that you will absolutely develop cancer. Being forewarned is forearmed. What this means is that you should immediately take all possible steps to reduce your risk from outside factors. Although you cannot control your genetic inheritance, you can incorporate preventive measures into your lifestyle.

Geopathogenic Zones

EARTH DISTURBANCES - What exactly are *geopathogenic* zones, probably a new term to most, if not all, of the American public. An examination of the word itself provides the explanation. *Geo* comes from the Greek and means 'the earth.' *Pathogenic* is defined as 'disease producing.' *What?* Are there then certain zones of the earth which foster the development of disease?

Unfortunately, the answer appears to be *yes*. As long ago as 1920, the world-renowned German surgeon and oncologist Dr. Sauerbruch advised his cancer patients not to return to their homes if they were in a geopathogenic zone. Research into the possibility of low-frequency electrical disturbances deep the earth increasing the risk of cancer to those who live in the vicinity began seriously over twenty years ago by Dr. Ernst Hartmann of Eberbach, Germany.

In the beginning, Dr. Hartmann's theory was ridiculed by orthodox medicine, and is still today rejected by most cancer authorities. But science has now determined that even a very weak electromagnetic pulse (between 5 and 25 Hz) can produce cancer cells. These extremely low frequencies (ELF) are active in geopathogenic zones. The major cause of these harmful ELF is the underground water flowing beneath the surface of the earth. The veins and arteries carrying the life-sustaining water supplies of the world produce these dangerous low frequencies, now known to cause the development of cancer in those living above them.

Further documentation comes from Dr. Nieper who reports the following as a result of his own research and continuing observation of the cancer victims he himself treats: "According to studies I initiated, at least 92 percent of all the cancer patients I examined have remained for long time periods - expecially with respect to their sleeping place - in geopathogenic zones. In my opinion, it is essential that tumor patients, as well as patients suffering from multiple sclerosis, be apprised of this information and depart geopathogenic zones."

There are certain manufactured devices avilable which are purported to *shield* the user from the damaging effects of the geopathogenic zones. Shielding devices are not effective. However, there are some devices which can, but only in part, *neutralize* the harmful ELF. One such device, called the 'North-South Rectifier,' is manufactured by the Henry Weber Company, Switzerland and another comes from Oberbach in Germany. At this writing, no effective ELF neutralizing devices are available in the U.S.

Electrical Fields

FRIEND TURNED FOE - Substantiating even further the harmful effect of certain electrical fields is the fact that persons working in electric transformer stations have a higher incidence of leukemia. Research originating at the University of Colorado corroborates the suspicion that people living in the vicinity of powerful electric mains suffer a higher incidence of cancer than the general population.

Another factor which is not well-known in the U.S. is the damaging effect of alternating current. How many of us sleep under electric blankets and expose ourselves nightly to ELF waves? Probably even more of us use an electric heating pad or massage unit to soothe aching muscles from time to time. *Don't*.

According to German studies, the alternating current generated by electric blankets, heating pads, massage units, and the like radiates from these commonly used items and inactivates the body's electrostatic filtering system which normally keeps the urinary tract passages bacteria-free.

Experienced (and aware) oncologists have observed that from the end of August until the first cold frosty nights of the winter season, the body's immune defense capacity is reduced by up to 30 percent. There is a documented and dramatic increase in the rate of growth of any malignancy in the body during this time of year. Around August 28th, the planets in the solar system pass through a dense system of magnetic fields. It is theorized that certain electromagnetic factors thus created contribute to a drop in the body's defense mechanisms. This effect continues until the planets move on in early January.

During the damp months of autumn and continuing until the first hard freeze of winter, any mother will tell you that her family is more subject to sore throats, coughs, colds, and flu. This phenomenon, long recognized, is at least partially due to the fact that the first freeze destroys airborne bacteria. However, now that science has determined that the immune system is not working at full capacity during the planetary configurations that occur during this period, researchers are taking a hard look at the possibility that electromagnetic pulses reaching the earth should figure into their calculations.

TEMPERATURE CONTROL - Another comfort of modern

technology which can become a potential health hazard is the American practice of turning up the thermostat. Of particular importance to all of us, especially cancer patients, is the news that experiments have shown that the body's immune defense system becomes sluggish and its efficiency drops drastically at temperatures over approximately 64.5 degrees F. (18 degrees C.).

Perhaps my readiness to accept the effects of the planets on man stems from learning the proper phases of the moon for planting from my grandfather. Or perhaps it's the memory of my grandmother and her unwavering belief in the importance of assisting the body through natural dietary means to work at optimum efficiency. But I can't help but observe that orthodox medicine seems determined to alter chemically (or cut out) rather than assist naturally by recommending the proper foods and supplements which are known to strengthen the body's immune defenses.

If some of this information is new to you, we invite you to consi-consider it carefully and incorporate whatever seems good and logical into your own lifestyle. Many of the preventive measures suggested are both inexpensive and simple. For instance, by merely adding carrot juice to your daily regimen, you will be providing your body with beta-carotene, an incredibly powerful cancer preventive.

I'll drink a toast to your health tomorrow morning at breakfast with my morning carrot juice! I recommend it highly.

EDITOR'S NOTE - The material in this chapter is a prepublication release and has been excerpted from a new in-depth book on cancer entitled *How to Fight Cancer & Win* (Fischer Publishing Company, Canfield, Ohio 44406), still in manuscript form. The author believes that this information could be of such vital importance to the American public that it should be made available immediately and not held pending future publication.

The World Famous

Dr. Rinse Formula

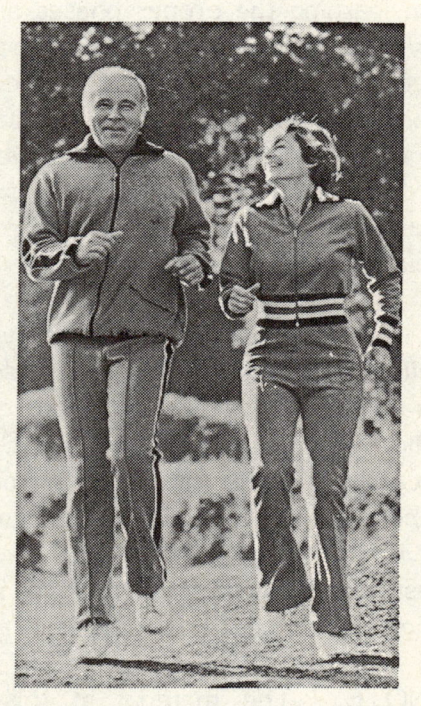

The amazing formula, developed by Dr. Rinse for his personal use after an incapacitating heart attack, has overcome heart disease in tens of thousands of individuals around the world. Empirical evidence in the form of testimonials from grateful users shows the Dr. Rinse Formula not only aids in the fight against cardiovascular and circulatory problems by cleaning out arteries clogged with cholesterol, but can reduce high blood pressure and even eases the pain of arthritis.

CHAPTER 18

Jacobus Rinse, Ph.D. The Man Himself

Luke 4:23 "Physician, heal thyself"

I became personally acquainted with Jacobus Rinse one crisp Sunday afternoon in the middle of his vast acreage in a remote corner of Vermont. My wife and I motored up from our home to have dinner at his invitation. We drove leisurely, thoroughly enjoying our passage through the rolling hills of Ohio, ablaze with the changing colors of autumn, up through the majestic mountains of Pennsylvania crowned with snow-caps and wreathed with hazy clouds of snow.

Following the good doctor's excellent directions, we finally reached the Rinse holdings and turned into the lane. As we drove down what has to be the longest "driveway" I ever traveled, we heard the sound of a chain-saw echoing across the river. As we continued driving down the lane, the sound got louder and we were busy looking around trying to spot the operator through the trees when the saw noise stopped.

Suddenly, coming across the river toward the road, there appeared Dr. Jacobus Rinse. I stopped the car and walked eagerly to greet him. I found it hard to believe this alert, vigorous man coming toward me with the welcoming smile was 84 years old. His stride was that of a much younger man and the chain-saw in his hand testified to his afternoon's occupation. "Just clearing out some dead wood," he explained. "I was cutting it into lengths to fit the fireplace and stacking it into cords."

After a very pleasant and convivial meal, I expressed my surprise and complimented him on his excellent physical condition. Even though I had read his published works and many of the articles written about him, I still was amazed to think he had transformed himself from a semi-invalid who, according to his medical prognosis, should have been dead long ago, into the dynamo seated before me.

He chuckled a little and told us a bit about his schedule. On many occasions, he said, he climbs into his old Volkswagen and makes the four-hour trip down to New York City in his capacity as chemical consultant. Upon arriving in the city, he may give a lecture, attend a luncheon or participate in a meeting. Without staying overnight or pausing to rest, he then climbs into the VW and makes the four-hour return trip. Dr. Rinse regularly works until 2:00 in the morning and boasts, in his words, "a heart as sound as a child's."

Although many people are unaware of it, the Dr. Rinse Formula he developed, and which has helped so many overcome their health problems, brings him no income. This remarkable man has no commercial interest in the preparation and accepts no remuneration whatsoever. It is strictly an altruistic effort. Dr. Jacobus Rinse is a benefactor of mankind and, as a healer, knows no peer.

When asked if he had any secrets, he smiled in reply. "No secrets. Proper nutrition, suitable exercise and my formula, that's all." Dr. Rinse says emphatically, "Anyone can have the same results."

In The Beginning

Thirty-four years ago, after suffering his first heart attack at the age of 51, Dr. Jacobus Rinse was told he had ten years to live—

provided he restricted all physical activity and took his prescribed medications daily. Remembering the sharp pain and agonizing vice-like constriction of the chest he experienced during his heart seizure, which followed an unusually active weekend clearing the land where his new house was to stand, Dr. Rinse resolved to follow the orders of his cardiologist to the letter. With his very life at stake, he had too much to lose to take any chances whatsoever. His life as a virtual invalid began.

Born and educated in Holland and holding a doctorate in physical chemistry, Dr. Rinse couldn't understand what factors had combined to create his heart condition. As a textbook case, he didn't fit. By medical standards, he should not have been a candidate for early heart problems. He knew that individuals at risk usually have a family history of heart disease, that many smoke, and that most are over-weight and eat a diet high in cholesterol. Dr. Rinse was the first member of his family to experience a heart attack, had never smoked and watched his diet, virtually eliminating foods targeted as high in cholesterol, such as eggs, butter, most dairy products and fatty meats. Other contributing factors to heart disease are thought to include physical strain to the breaking point and emotional stress or excitement continuing over a period of time. He examined his life and found these criteria did not apply to him either.

Yet, in spite of his healthy lifestyle, his angina attack was the very real result of an atherosclerotic condition characterized by cholesterol-clogged arteries. Popping nitroglycerin pellets, sometimes as often as every fifteen or thirty minutes, to open up the constricted arteries which caused his heart to spasm painfully, was not to his liking. Dr. Rinse explains, "I was not satisfied to make use of these small pellets for the rest of my life - even if it was only to be 10 years."

As a practicing research chemist, Dr. Rinse determined to change his body chemistry and reverse his prognosis. He started investigating natural foods thought to protect against cholesterol buildup and began eating raw foods rich in fat-liquifying enzymes. From 1951 when he suffered his first heart failure until 1957, he lived on raw fruits, raw vegetables, raw herring, raw meat, raw eggs and yogurt. He began taking 1000 mg of Vitamin C (ascorbic acid) daily and a multivitamin tablet. Being aware of the research of Evan Shute, M.D. and Wilfrid E. Shute, M.D. of Ontario, Canada who successfully treated many heart patients with Vitamin E, he determined to follow their recommendations and began taking 200 mg of Vitamin E after meals.

During this period, Dr. Rinse relates that the one single supplement he felt helped him best tolerate increased physical activity was *garlic*. Talking of the rigid regimen he set for himself and followed without deviation for six long years, Dr. Rinse now says, "By avoiding overly strenuous exercise, I managed to live a more or less normal life."

However, his satisfactions were few and in 1957, he experienced another excruciating attack, lasting an agonizing hour this time.

He suffered almost constant spasms of angina pain, in spite of his medication. His heart rate rose an alarming 50 beats and he was slow to recover after the slightest amount of exercise. It was beginning to appear the medical experts were right after all.

With six years of his precious projected ten gone, Dr. Rinse refused to be conquered and began his serious research all over again. There had to be a key.

Certain scientific tests conducted on laboratory animals with chemically-induced high cholesterol levels came to his attention. This research indicated that the substance *lecithin*, derived from soybeans, could actually dissolve cholesterol. In addition, *safflower oil* was shown to contain precisely the polyunsaturated fatty acids needed to reduce cholesterol to a liquid state. Could it be possible that a combination of lecithin and safflower oil would conquer atherosclerosis in humans and clear clogged arteries? Dr. Rinse decided to find out, using himself as a guinea pig.

Along with his other supplements, he began to take one tablespoon each of lecithin and safflower oil daily. Incredible as it may sound, in only a *few days*, he began to feel the difference as his body responded.

Dr. Rinse reported, "My angina pains ceased. My galloping pulse rate decreased slightly, but noticeably. Excellent results began to appear within a few days." After three months of continued use, his angina symptoms totally disappeared, even after exercise. The chemist in him attributed his improvement to the lecithin and safflower oil.

One short year later, his physical activity now encompassing even heavy outside work, his condition appeared completely cured. Dr. Rinse explained, "I am convinced the food supplement I developed is both a preventive and cure for atherosclerosis. I have had no recurrence of angina or other diseases. It seems the atherosclerotic plaques which had been narrowing my arteries to cause heart failure have been reversed."

Judging from his extraordinary health at 84 years of age, Dr. Jacobus Rinse was completely correct. He has personally conquered one of the major killers of our time.

The Dr. Rinse Formula - A Personal Account

Recently, my mother-in-law, 69, frail, with a weak heart, suffering from atherosclerosis and angina pain, crippled and all but incapacitated by arthritis and osteoporosis, took it into her sweet stubborn head to leave her native Bavaria and come to the United States to visit us. My wife was frantic with worry over her condition and certain the trip would end with our having to put her in a hospital. She prayed only that it wouldn't happen en route, with Nan-Nan being rushed on an emergency basis to a hospital in some distant city.

We tried every which way to change Nan-Nan's mind, including several *very* long-distance phone calls, but it didn't matter to her that we had a trip scheduled to see her the coming autumn and offered to escort her back with us; it didn't matter to her that her health really wasn't up to such a long trip and she refused to confront the possibility of a fall which could result in broken bones already weakened by her osteoporosis.

Osteoporosis is a very common condition in the elderly, especially those living alone. It is caused by a disturbance of the body's metabolism resulting from a deficiency of certain nutrients and minerals (primarily calcium), usually present in an adequate diet. But, like many senior citizens, Nan-Nan's family had scattered. With no one to cook for but herself, we were sure she had lost interest in food and no longer bothered to serve herself a balanced meal. Without the elements they need to keep strong, bone mass and density decrease, the bone becomes honeycombed with too much air space and osteoporosis progresses rapidly. Such bones are brittle, fragile and break very easily.

Nan-Nan had already undergone two separate operations for joint replacement when her brittle bones had snapped and would not heal. She was in constant pain from angina and the osteoporosis, and favored her right side when she walked, creating a back problem as well.

Nan-Nan's angina attacks required strong medication to bring the pain to bearable levels. The coronary insufficiency she labored under was caused by an advanced case of atherosclerosis, commonly called "hardening of the arteries," often making her short of breath as her heart labored to send oxygenated blood where it was needed. With the blood flow to her heart slowed by constricted and ever-narrowing blood vessels, she was a prime candidate for a heart attack, stroke or other degenerative condition - all of which come from atherosclerosis.

Add to that the swollen joints and nodules of the arthritis that cruelly curled her hands and sent pains shooting through her body and you can well understand why we were worried about Nan-Nan making such a long trip alone.

Always indomitable, Nan-Nan let us know she was determined to come alone *now* - and that's exactly what she did. The relief was evident on my wife's face when we met the plane and she could finally put her arms around the tiny hobbling figure and support her to the car. Her face was gray with the fatigue of the long flight, but we got her home and I tucked her up warm and cozy while my wife went to fetch a cup of herb tea and honey for all of us.

Leaving them to chat a little, I took my tea downstairs to my favorite chair and began to think seriously about Nan-Nan's medical problems. Certainly it was going to be easy to make sure she had an adequate diet while she was with us, but she refused to leave her home-place and live with any of her children. What would happen to her health when she went back home? What single one thing could we do for her that was simple and easy enough for her to continue when she returned to Bavaria? What could we do in the four short months of her visit that would make enough difference in the way she felt so that she would *want* to continue it herself? Suddenly it came to me! Nan-Nan would join us in taking the *Dr. Rinse Formula breakfast-mash* every day.

Two years before when I was entering my 50s, I found I was slowing down and I didn't like it. I had always followed what are generally considered good health practices and enjoyed robust good health for the whole of my life, but I suddenly found myself puffing going up the stairs and continually fell asleep after dinner. Although there wasn't anything I could really put my finger on, except shortness-of-breath and lack of energy, I took myself to the doctor. He joked I was "just getting old," but put me through a complete battery of tests. He found my cholesterol levels were elevated above the normal range and talked to me about "hardening of the arteries" and what medical problems atherosclerosis could create.

In 1983, I had presented "The Dr. Rinse Formula" to my readers. I was personally very impressed with the good doctor and his natural nutritional almost-miraculous cures of atherosclerosis, high (and low) blood pressure, arthritis, bursitis, phlebitis, angina and more. I recalled such a flood of letters from grateful individuals testifying joyously to their renewed well-being and health after taking Dr. Rinse's Formula, it created a happy problem - that of selecting just a few to exerpt for publication! The very thing for me, I thought to myself.

From that time on, my wife and I began taking Dr. Rinse's breakfast-mash religiously. My cholesterol reading fell dramatically and I have the boundless energy of a child again. My wife glows and the twinges of early arthritis she was experiencing have vanished. Apparently we had caught ourselves in time, but what about Nan-Nan? Could Dr. Rinse's Formula help such a diversity of medical problems all concentrated in one frail old body?

YES! The very next morning, with a little urging from my wife, Nan-Nan downed her portion of Dr. Rinse's Formula and dutifully took the alfalfa tablets I laid out for her. Although her problems were of very long-standing, I am absolutely delighted to report that within just two weeks, changes in her condition were noticeable. Her breathing was no longer labored and she seemed to be getting around more comfortably. Within two short months, she was able to help around the house - and enjoyed it thoroughly. By the time she left to return home after four months with us, she was freely moving her fingers without pain for the first time in eight years, thanks to the Rinse Formula and the alfalfa tablets!

It is impossible to fully describe the dramatic changes Dr. Rinse's Formula worked for Nan-Nan. We brought home a fragile, stooped old lady suffering from a seemingly impossible conglomeration of ills and sent home a relatively spry happy oldster looking forward to life again! Her last letter says she is doing marvelously and confirms she will never be without her breakfast-mash. I, for one, am not surprised! Chalk up another victory for Dr. Rinse.

Nutrition For a Healthy Heart

WHY THE RINSE FORMULA WORKS - According to the most recent Vital Statistics report as tabulated and compiled by the United States government, nearly three-quarters of American deaths can be traced to four causes: cancer, stroke, accident and *heart disease*. The National Center for Health Statistics report for the year 1982 shows that 326 persons died of heart disease out of every 100,000 Americans that year, making heart disease the major killer of our civilization. Orthodox medical treatment, notably the attempt to regulate serum cholesterol levels, does not appear able to stem the tide.

IS CHOLESTEROL THE CULPRIT? - Cholesterol is an organic compound of the steroid family and occurs either free or as esters of fatty acids in practically all animal tissues. *Cholesterol is the raw material from which the body produces bile acids, steroid hormones and provitamin D3.* Cholesterol makes up about 3/10th of one percent of weight in the average person. It isn't the cholesterol in the blood that creates the problem, it's whether or not the body has the other materials needed to process it properly.

ATHEROSCLEROSIS - WHAT IS IT? - The old-fashioned term *hardening of the arteries* says it all. If atherosclerotic plaques injure the artery lining, cholesterol and other fats build up on the arterial walls narrowing the passageway and impeding the flow of oxygenated blood. When this happens, the individual is at risk and will most likely suffer a heart attack, stroke or phlebitis. Because it has been clinically determined that an excessive amount of cholesterol in the blood can cause atherosclerosis, medical science has targeted cholesterol as a major factor in heart disease.

CAN CHOLESTEROL BE CONTROLLED BY DIET? - Science has shown that the amount of cholesterol consumed in the daily diet does not determine the amount of serum cholesterol levels in the blood. The body itself can manufacture up to about 1.5 grams of cholesterol per day. *If cholesterol in the diet is reduced, the body simply increases its manufacture.* Research has shown that diets low in cholesterol are often ineffective in reducing serum cholesterol levels.

What about cholesterol-lowering drugs? A study conducted with 8,000 heart patients on the so-called cholesterol-lowering drugs over a seven year period of time did not result in a lowering of the projected death rate. The cost of this experimental investigation was over forty million dollars and none of the drugs showed a favorable influence on the death rate.

Many authorities are now taking a second look at the theory which forbids heart patients or those considered at risk of heart disease the dietary delights of such highly nutritious and common foods as butter, milk, eggs, beef and so on. The basis for this theory is the fact that these foods contain cholesterol-producing saturated animal fats. However, they all *also* contain more than enough *high-density lipoproteins* (HDL) to keep cholesterol in a liquid state.

WHAT ARE "LIPO-PROTEINS?" - Lipoproteins are fat-protein molecules which either carry cholesterol to the tissues, or remove cholesterol from the tissues. It is the *low-density lipoproteins* (LDL) which carry cholesterol *to* the tissues and the *high-density lipoproteins* (HDL) which dissolve and carry cholesterol *away* from the tissues. It has been determined that an important indicator of the possibility of a heart attack is actually the ratio of HDL to LDL. It is therefore desirable to have a high HDL and low LDL ratio.

LECITHIN & LINOLEIC - THE FRIENDLY FATS -Cholesterol can be dissolved in the blood only in the presence of linoleate-lecithin. Because the melting point of cholesterol is 300 degrees F., it is deposited on arterial walls as a insoluble substance at the normal body temperature of 98.6 degrees. However, with the saturated fatty acids of lecithin present, the melting point of cholesterol is reduced to 180 degrees F., still insoluble at body temperature. When linoleate oil is added, the melting point of cholesterol is brought down to 32 degrees F., well below normal body temperature. In a liquid state, cholesterol is not deposited on arterial walls.

A study examining 900 men for atherosclerosis conclusively showed that all *individuals with more than 36% lecithin in their blood had no atherosclerosis*. Individuals with 34% or less lecithin showed evidence of the disease. Because HDL dissolves cholesterol, there is a resulting absence of atherosclerotic plaque, and existing deposits are carried away as well.

KIDS & CHOLESTEROL - Researchers at the University of Cincinnati are saying that it might not be a bad idea to monitor cholesterol levels in children. The experts say that high cholesterol levels established in early years and allowed to progress unchecked set the stage for heart disease as the child matures.

In support of this premise, the scientists cite findings from autopsies performed on American soldiers killed in the Korean War. Most of these young men were around twenty years of age, but the surprise was that a great many of them had serious atherosclerotic plaque buildup in their arteries. Healthy young men in their twenties are not usually considered at risk of heart disease.

A cholesterol level of 185 in children and young people aged two to nineteen appears to put them in the high risk category. At least one of the medical doctors involved in this new area of research says that he "would feel comfortable aiming for a cholesterol count of around 160." The researchers note that, as for adults, just monitoring cholesterol levels isn't enough. It's also important to take a reading of the child's HDL count to determine just how the body is handling cholesterol.

THE RINSE FORMULA contains both lecithin and raw sunflower seeds, which provide the necessary linoleate oil.

BREWER'S YEAST & WHEAT GERM - Both Brewer's yeast and wheat germ are particularly good sources of the B vitamins, including inositol and choline. If the body is deficient in these important vitamins, lecithin cannot be produced in adequate amounts. Even a mild deficiency of choline has been shown to decrease the amount of lecithin in the blood and causes less of the cholesterol passing through the liver to be converted into bile. A lack of choline slows down the use of cholesterol in the tissues and encourages heavy fatty deposits in the arteries.

A study conducted with patients recovering from heart attacks confirmed that when choline and inositol were supplemented in the diet, the size of the cholesterol particles and amount of fat in the blood decreased quickly. Within two months, serum cholesterol levels were normal. It must be pointed out that cholesterol cannot be reduced by choline and/or inositol alone, but must be accompanied by lecithin. In addition, lecithin cannot be synthesized in the body without enzymes containing Vitamin B6. These important enzymes, in turn, are active only if magnesium is present.

THE RINSE FORMULA contains debittered Brewer's yeast and wheat germ, both excellent natural sources of choline, inositol and B6.

VITAMIN B6 (PYRIDOXINE) - A low Vitamin B6 level is often characterized by moodiness (or depression if B6 deficiency is severe), nervousness, a feeling of weakness, a lack of energy, water retention and even the inability to remember dreams. Deficiency of B6 often occurs in individuals with a family history of diabetes, celiac disease and hypoglycemia. Some prescription drugs, gastrointestinal disease and radiation therapy deplete the body's stores of B6.

Vitamin B6 is required by the body as a co-enzyme and in metabolic function. It plays a part in protecting the sheath around our nerves and must be present for the body to make efficient use of proteins and amino acids. As does Vitamin C, Vitamin B6 assists in converting amino acids to neurotransmitters (the means brain cells use to communicate with each other). It has been reported to relieve the nausea caused by radiation sickness and the typical morning-sickness of pregnancy. Vitamin B6 has been successfully used in the clinical treatment of arthritis and is reported to reduce the pain and swelling of joints thickened by this disease.

A deficiency of Vitamin B6 has been shown to lead to the development of atherosclerotic plaque. Researchers working under the auspices of MIT found a deficiency of this vital vitamin, especially in conjunction with a high protein diet, can actually cause atherosclerosis. The body converts methionine (an antioxidant amino acid) into homocysteine (an oxidant) which requires B6 to produce cystothionine (a helpful antioxidant). If your diet contains a lot of cooked meat, which produces an excess of methionine, and is also lacking in B6, chances are you are inviting cardiovascular disease.

On the bright side, supplementing the diet with B6 not only assures you are supplying an important nutrient to your heart, but researchers believe B6 can increase energy levels, improve your resistance to stress and may even protect your normal emotional health.

THE RINSE FORMULA provides a healthy measure of Vitamin B6 (pyridoxine), naturally occurring in two important ingredients (wheat germ and yeast). Note: this may be the reason why so many arthritics on the Rinse Formula report improvement in their condition as well.

MAGNESIUM - The need for magnesium supplements is magnified by a prolonged siege of diarrhea, a liquid postoperative (or weight-loss) diet, the use of diuretics and the consumption of large amounts of alcohol. A magnesium deficiency often shows itself in irritability, nervousness, foot and leg cramps, muscular weakness - and an irregular heart beat.

An important point to note is that even when Vitamin B6 is present in adequate amounts, a deficiency of magnesium prevents lecithin from forming and slows down the body's use of fats and cholesterol. Research indicates that heart patients given magnesium as a supplement made dramatic improvement and serum cholesterol levels were drastically reduced in just one month.

When serum cholesterol levels are high, the need for magnesium is critical. In a laboratory experiment, rats fed hydrogenated fat and raw cholesterol required sixteen times more magnesium than rats fed a normal diet. When their diet was supplemented with adequate magnesium, however, the rats did not develop atherosclerosis. Even after the arteries were heavily clogged with fatty deposits, adequate magnesium caused cholesterol levels to drop to normal range and the arteries cleared and became healthy.

Further, adequate magnesium levels are shown to fight stress, help maintain normal muscle contraction ability and aid in the body's adaption to cold. Note: In areas of the country where "soft" water lacking in many minerals exists, science has documented higher magnesium deficiencies.

THE RINSE FORMULA contains the appropriate amount of magnesium needed for heart health.

BONEMEAL (DICALCIUM PHOSPHATE) — Although many foods in the normal diet contain phosphorous, and a lack of phosphorus is rare, calcium is supplied only by various forms of milk. Contrary to popular opinion, even cheeses (unless made with sweet milk) contain little calcium. Authorities believe 2 grams of calcium should be taken daily by the average adult. Unfortunately, because a quart of milk (whole, buttermilk, yogurt, acidophilus) supplies only 1 gram, supplementation is highly desirable for optimum functioning.

A calcium deficiency creates a susceptibility to bone fractures, promotes lower-back pain, a softening of the bones and sets the stage for periodontal disease. If you are on a bed-rest program, are in an orthopedic cast and can't (or don't) exercise, chances are you need additional calcium in your diet. A high-flouride intake, high-protein diets, emotional stress and hard work in high temperatures increase the body's need for calcium. It has long been recognized that nursing mothers and pregnant or menopausal women require extra calcium in their diet.

THE RINSE FORMULA contains the necessary amount of dicalcium phosphate in bonemeal form.

VITAMIN C (ASCORBIC ACID) — Never underestimate the importance of Vitamin C. Those who bruise easily, have excessive dental problems (including spongy bleeding gums), or who suffer tiny hemorrhages of the blood vessels under the skin, commonly known as "spider" veins, may be exhibiting a need for Vitamin C supplementation. An increased need has also been demonstrated in smokers, diabetics, the elderly, allergy victims and individuals under stress.

All animals, including man, must have Vitamin C to survive. Many animals produce Vitamin C in their liver or adrenals, but man lacks the enzyme required in the manufacturing process and must replenish his supply either by a good diet of fresh foods or by supplementation. Vitamin C is needed to guard the brain and spinal cord from free radicals, for connective tissue (collagen) synthesis, for efficient metabolism of fats and carbohydrates, to produce neurotransmitters and for the maintenance of our all-important immune system.

Vitamin C acts as a natural antibiotic, promotes healing, helps maintain healthy gums, keeps the body cooler during exercise, increases energy levels and fights the effects of stress. Many researchers believe Vitamin C offers protection against the common cold and may yet prove to be the answer to the flu.

Vitamin C is also an important ingredient in the management of cholesterol. Research has determined that when HDL and cholesterol reach the liver together, HDL is removed and decomposes. In the presence of Vitamin C, the cholesterol is then converted into bile acids and never reaches the arteries. It passes into the duodenum (portion of the small intestine) where it aids in the emulsification and absorption of fats. As an aid to reduction of serum cholesterol, Vitamin C taken by mouth has been shown to reduce levels of cholesterol in the blood by 35 to 40%.

THE RINSE FORMULA contains the right amount of Vitamin C needed daily by man, both as an aid to cholesterol management and for life.

VITAMIN E (D-ALPHA TOCOPHEROL) - If you suffer from hot flashes, skin problems, muscle cramping, and hands and feet which are always cold (signaling a circulatory problem resulting in insufficient blood flow to the extremities) your body may be trying to tell you something. These are all common symptoms of Vitamin E deficiency.

In addition, Vitamin E is the body's most important fat soluble antioxidant. It protects lipids (fats) in our body from uncontrolled oxidation and free radicals. Oxidation can cause cancer, induce blood clots resulting in heart attack or stroke, and can damage the element in our cells which controls growth, development and aging. Megadosage levels of Vitamin E have been shown to increase resistance to cancer, bacterial and viral infections, stroke, arthritis, heart attack and environmental pollution.

Vitamin E provides substantial protection against heart attacks by preventing abnormal clot formation. Research has shown Vitamin E slows the formation time for abnormal clotting and even prolongs the clotting time of recalcified human plasma. This effect can reduce the incidence of coronary thrombosis in which a clot breaks loose and travels to the heart, resulting in a heart attack. In the literature of the world's medical community, there are over 130 papers supporting the use of Vitamin E in treating and overcoming heart disease.

Vitamin E not only acts as an antioxidant, but promotes a healthy circulatory system, fights environmental toxins and boosts the immune system. Note: Science has determined those who live or work in areas where chemical or environmental pollutants are present in high concentrations have an increased need for Vitamin E.

THE RINSE FORMULA contains Vitamin E in its pure form and also as an element present in wheat germ.

ZINC - A serious zinc deficiency often results in a loss (or diminishing) of the taste sense, usually accompanied by a loss of appetite and the sense of smell. A lack of zinc has also been linked to prostate problems in men over 40 and may contribute to infertility and even diabetes. Low levels of zinc have been shown to slow wound healing and result in a poor resistance to infections as well.

For heart health, zinc is an important mineral which functions as an antioxidant to protect the cell membranes against free radical damage. Science has determined free radical activity increases when inadequate oxygen is supplied to the tissues. Many heart attacks and most strokes can be attributed to poor oxygenation of the blood. Free radical damage often occurs in atherosclerosis because of insufficient circulation. Zinc is one of the specific nutrients which protects the immune system.

THE RINSE FORMULA contains the appropriate amount of zinc, an important antioxidant.

Dr. Rinse's files are bulging with letters and case histories of people from all over the world who have used his nutrient formula to cure cardiovascular disease. Dr. Rinse says, "I developed this formula during seven years of trial and error. Now, because of the overwhelming bio-chemical evidence in its support and the success with its use, which many hundreds of people in the United States and Europe have reported, I believe strongly in this food supplement formulation I've evolved."

Dr. Rinse's Formula Praised by Many
Here's a Small Sampling from our Files

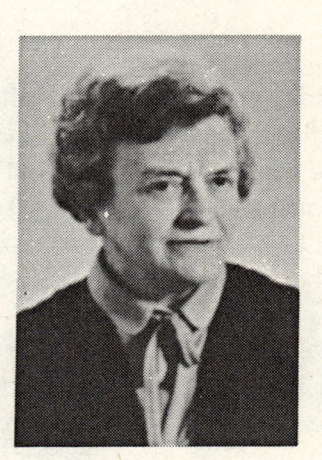

Mrs. Elizabeth Bouse
Housewife
Trenton, New Jersey

Mrs. Bouse, 70 years old, tells us she had been afflicted with swelling of her hands and knuckles and was unable to do any housework for many years. Atherosclerosis and arthritis affected both her knees so severely she was barely able to move around. Even daily chores were beyond her. When a friend told her about it, Mrs. Bouse started taking the Dr. Rinse Formula and three alfalfa tablets three times daily. Her condition began to improve in just two weeks. After two more weeks, her fingers became more flexible and she lost the stiffness in her knees. She was very happy to be able to move around more freely and now rejoices in being able to do her own housework again! After three months on the Dr. Rinse diet, all her symptoms disappeared and she was able to do her daily chores without pain for the first time in many, many years. Mrs. Bouse's doctor was amazed at her improvement and he's now recommending this diet to his patients with similar conditions!

Mrs. Trudy Wein
Billings, Montana

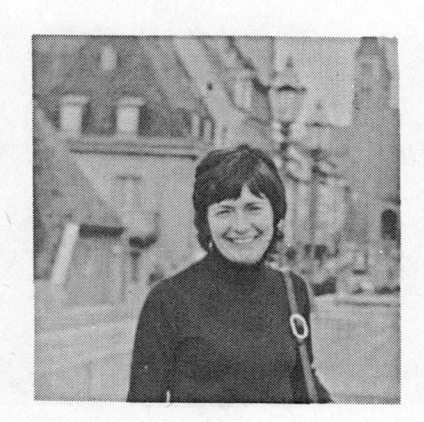

When I turned 40, my doctor put me on medication for various disorders, such as atherosclerosis, arthritis and hypoglycemia (low blood sugar). My blood pressure was always very low and I suffered from cold hands and feet for many years. My fingers and toes felt numb most of the time, except when the arthritic pain caused my fingers to swell and hurt. I took a strong medication which helped my condition somewhat, but at the same time, I became very dizzy, couldn't sleep, had migraine headaches and a sinus condition. A friend of mine read your book and told me about the incredible results she had experienced just by taking the Dr. Rinse breakfast mash. She convinced me. After only a month, I could see the first signs of improvement myself. I'm 45 now and have been using the Dr. Rinse formula for six months. All my symptoms have completely vanished! I can't believe the difference. I can run up the stairs without puffing, my hands and feet are always warm, and my doctor discontinued my medication. Even my cholesterol level is normal. I'm very thankful for this improvement. My doctor now gives me a clean and perfect bill of health. I'm full of energy and everyone thinks I look about ten years younger!

Professor Dr.
Armin
Hoelscher
Chemist and
Pharmacist,
Retired
St. Petersburg,
Florida

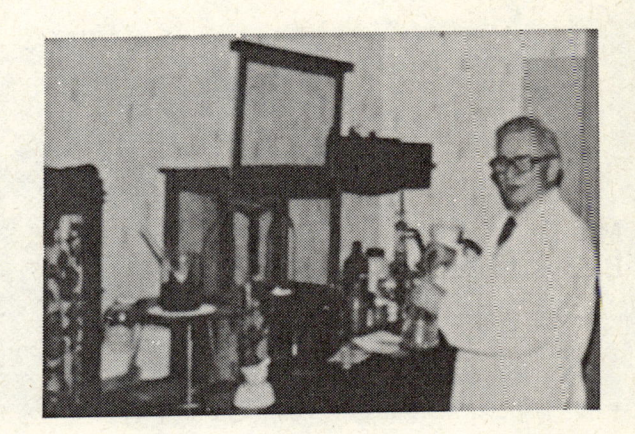

This 84-year old professional man had severe angina, heart problems, poor blood circulation, very low blood pressure and a high cholesterol level, plus other serious cardiovascular-related ailments. Dr. Hoelscher was unable to walk more than a few hundred yards without stopping frequently to catch his breath. He suffered an artery blockage in his lower right extremities, causing him severe pain. He was forced to drag his right leg as he walked. He was on Lanicor for many years to stabilize his failing heart. After using the Dr. Rinse Formula for just four weeks, he wrote us to say he could feel his symptoms slowly diminishing. After three months on the Dr. Rinse mash, the Professor was able to breathe more freely, could walk up steps without problems and even resumed his morning walks for the first time in many years. After two more months on the mash, Dr. Hoelscher wrote again to tell us of his joy at being able to walk up to two miles daily and do some vigorous exercise and heavy outdoor work. We were especially pleased to hear from this scientist. As a pharmacist and chemist, he was skeptical at first, but is now convinced. What all his other medications were unable to do, the all-natural Dr. Rinse Formula accomplished by providing him all the essentials he needed to stabilize his health!

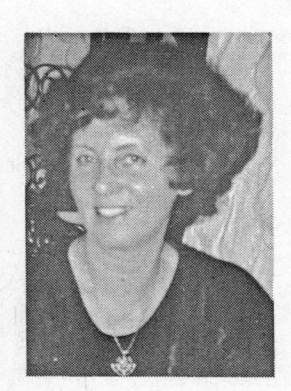

Maria Nobles
Dress Shop Owner
Tampa, Florida

Although I'm in my early fifties, I have always enjoyed very good health. When I broke my ankle last year, my doctor suggested that I have a thorough physical examination. I didn't want to bother, but my husband told the doctor that I sometimes had trouble breathing and had fainted several times. When the doctor heard this, he insisted on a complete series of tests. He discovered that I had seriously elevated levels of cholesterol and triglycerides and explained that my breathing difficulties and fainting spells were caused by clogged arteries leading to impaired circulation. My blood wasn't transporting sufficient oxygen to my brain. He said I was at serious risk of having a major stroke or heart attack and put me on medication. These pills seemed to take away all my energy. I was so tired I could barely drag myself to my shop every day.

A friend told me her husband had had the same problem. I had trouble believing that because I know him to be very active and always busy. She said that the Dr. Rinse Formula had made a big difference in his health and gave me a copy of your book. She urged me to read about it and then try it. I can't tell you how happy I am that I took her good advice!

Since I've been taking the Dr. Rinse Formula every morning at breakfast, I've regained both my good disposition and my health has improved to the point where even my doctor says I don't need my prescribed medication any longer. He's amazed at how quickly I regained my good health by simply taking the Dr. Rinse Formula.

A.M.H.
Chemist
Borger, Texas

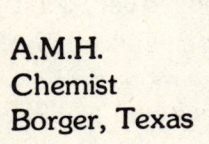

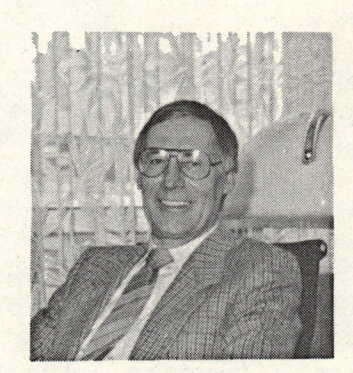

I am 60 years old and hold the equivalent to a major in biology from the University of Missouri. I was the Chief Chemist for Phillips Petroleum during my professional career and am now retired. After reading about Dr. Rinse, I started taking his formula in 1973 with about 2 teaspoons of soy lecithin granules and 1½ teaspoons of safflower oil each morning for breakfast. The mixture was supposed to keep cholesterol in solution so it would not form a slime in the blood vessel which could break loose and plug an artery. At this writing, I have cut back to a rounded teaspoon of lecithin and 1 teaspoon of oil.

After about two years on the Formula, my doctor asked me what I was doing. He said blood tests were like an 18-year old's! After my regular physical exam two years later, he again expressed amazement at my blood tests. After two more years on the breakfast-mash, I took a physical in Temple, Texas and they said the same!

This Formula is so good, it should be publicized to help humanity!

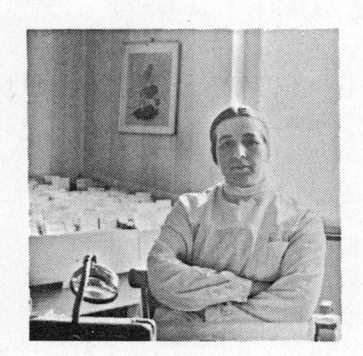

Elna Groth, N.D.
Naturopathic Physician
Austria

This naturally-oriented health-care professional writes: I'm using strictly homeopathic medicine to take care of my patients' health problems. But sometimes homeopathy doesn't give lasting results and I'm always searching for better treatment for my patients' ailments. While on vacation a few years ago in the U.S., I learned of the Dr. Rinse Formula and have since used it on many hundreds of my patients suffering health conditions that don't normally respond well to any medication. I have seen the most wonderful results with this mixture of vitamins in such cases as heart disease, angina and other coronary problems. Many of my patients afflicted with arthritis, gout, varicose veins, high cholesterol and even eye disorders, such as glaucoma, have responded favorably. I myself have been using Dr. Rinse's mash for almost two years. I must say I feel more energetic and positively rejuvenated! My blood pressure, always a problem, is now normalized.

Based on the incredible results I have seen in my patients and the studies on nutrition I have been doing, I feel this formula can overcome the hardships of disease and save many lives. The Dr. Rinse Formula may well be considered a universal health formula for many ailments. I can highly praise it from my own experience. Every person of middle-age should consider the Dr. Rinse mash daily. I believe it may ward off a lot of ailments that might otherwise occur. Dr. Rinse has developed a good, wholesome, natural preventive medicine of the finest kind.

The Dr. Rinse Formula

THE PROPORTIONS GIVEN BELOW WILL MAKE A 14-DAY SUPPLY

7 Tablespoons Lecithin granules
6 Tablespoons raw Wheat Germ
6 Tablespoons debittered Brewer's Yeast (powder or flakes)
6 Tablespoons Sunflower Seeds
6 teaspoons Bonemeal from a reliable source (powder or tablets)
6 Vitamin C tablets of 0.5 grams each
6 Vitamin E tablets (200 International Units total)

TO THESE INGREDIENTS, I ALSO ADD:

6 Tablespoons Bran Flakes (for better bowel movement)
6 teaspoons Kelp powder (or 6-12 Kelp tablets)
12 Zinc Oxide tablets of 10 mg each

All seeds or tablets should first be crushed in a blender.

Blend these ingredients well in a big bowl, stirring until the mixture is uniform. For improved health, take 1 to 2 Tablespoons of the Formula on a daily basis. To insure freshness and complete potency of all ingredients, I recommend you store your Dr. Rinse Formula in a closely covered jar in the refrigerator.

For my personal use, I also add a good dollop (about 1 Tablespoon) of raw, unheated unfiltered honey straight from a friendly neighbor's beehive. You may use molasses, if you prefer. The honey or molasses should be added at the time you swallow the mixture. My morning regimen also includes a good multi-vitamin/mineral tablet and three to five natural alfalfa tablets. When selecting your alfalfa tablets, be sure to secure them from a good reliable source. Shaklee is my choice.

As "heart-health" maintenance, we take 1 Tablespoon daily to create the catalytic effect we desire for our hearts. In case of heart disease, arthritis, rheumatism, osteoporosis, gout or combination-conditions, such as Nan-Nan suffered, be sure to take five or six alfalfa tablets three times daily. Alfalfa helps wash out toxins that have built up over the years and adds minerals needed by the body to repair damaged cell tissue.

We often take our portion of the Dr. Rinse breakfast-mash as a tasty addition to our morning cereal. As a change of pace, we sometimes use it to top yogurt or blend it into a high-protein shake. If you don't mind a somewhat "lumpy" drink, you may also stir it into any juice, such as grape, orange, pineapple or, my favorite, cranberry.

I want to add a word here about honey. Besides being a good natural "energizer," honey is one of nature's most powerful germ killers. Harmful bacteria cannot survive in raw honey. (Editor's note: It's the bee pollen particles suspended in the raw honey that makes it a germicide. See Chapter 13.) Primitive man made this discovery early on and used honey both as a sweet treat *and* as a salve to heal wounds. And, did you know that honey used as a sweetener doesn't result in the production of heavy body fat, as does refined sugar? Honey is delicious and digestible, as well as being nutritious. In fact, many nutrition experts consider honey a supplier of power for the heart muscle itself! If you prefer Dr. Rinse's Formula sweetened, you may add honey with a heavy hand and a clear conscience!

Once you start taking the Formula, don't be impatient! Although it is true some individuals seem to experience almost immediate relief, plan on allowing three months before the results become perceptible to you - and be pleasantly surprised if it happens sooner! After six months on the Formula, its therapeutic value will be quite apparent and you will surely be on your way to better all-around health. One final note: Authorities agree that restricting food to a low-fat diet is a good practice and will go a long way toward avoiding heart attacks, strokes and senility.

TIP: Even if you're not suffering from atherosclerosis, arthritis, hypertension (high blood pressure) or are not at risk of cardiovascular disease, I promise the Dr. Rinse Formula will improve the quality of your health and give you so much rip-roaring energy you'll feel like a frisky kid again!

CHAPTER 19

Conquering Depression & Handling Stress

Nutrients & Support Therapies That Work

A NATIONAL EPIDEMIC—Statistics show that over 20 million men and women, many of them teen-agers, are suffering from some sort of depressive disorder. Only about half of this number seek and find help. (One out of every ten prescriptions written by medical doctors in the U.S. is for one of the antidepressant drugs.) More than 250,000 victims diagnosed as suffering from clinical depression spend their lives in institutional facilities, and upwards of 20,000 depressives give up and manage to commit suicide every year.

Categorizing The Depressive State

NORMAL DEPRESSION—It is normal to be depressed at times in this imperfect world, but it is also normal to work through our bad feelings and regain our equilibrium. That's not what this chapter is all about. What we are discussing here are various abnormal depressive states that the individual cannot overcome alone.

SIMPLE DEPRESSION—A person in a state of simple depression goes about his daily affairs and continues near-normal functioning, but is obviously withdrawn and often appears miserable *without an apparent reason.*

CLINICAL DEPRESSION—In a severe or clinical depressive state, the individual is physically and mentally unable to function and is usually completely withdrawn from reality. Treatment is mandatory and hospitalization is common.

MANIC-DEPRESSION—A manic-depressive exhibits extreme variances in mood, with the depressive state occurring more often and lasting longer. In the euphoric phase of this condition, the manic-depressive typically exhibits abnormally high spirits and experiences a spurt of energy followed by an ever-deepening depression.

SEASONAL AFFECTIVE DISORDER—*SAD,* or Seasonal Affective Disorder, is a newly identified depressive state which afflicts certain individuals during the dark months of winter. Symptoms are the same as experienced in clinical depression, but are seasonal and disappear during summer. (An explanation of cause and the simple treatment of SAD occurs later in this chapter.)

The Symptoms of Depression

In a clinical depressive state, the symptoms typically exhibited are both physical and mental. Be on the alert for:
1. Complaints of constant fatigue, headaches, and/or stomach pains and cramps which cannot (or have not) been traced to a physical origin.
2. A weight loss or gain triggered by a lack of appetite or enormous need to eat continually, with alternating periods of diarrhea or constipation.

3. An abnormal need for sleep (or sudden periods of insomnia) and nightmares in which the individual continually experiences misfortune or tragedy.
4. Expressions of worthlessness and/or hopelessness; an expressed desire to "end it all." (It is *not* true that those who talk of suicide never actually do it.)
5. A state of deep depression occurring for no discernible reason which continues for a long period of time. Or, when related to a known situation (such as the death of a loved one), the individual does not progress through the normal stages of grief and depression.
6. A lack of interest in daily affairs, which may occur gradually over a period of time or appear quite suddenly with no warning. This phase commonly progresses to a complete withdrawal, resulting in:
7. The inability to function in the workplace, the home, or society in general.

The Cause Of Depression

EMOTIONAL—Psychiatrists and psychoanalysts proceed on the theory that a long-buried and suppressed trauma gives rise to depression. In some instances, this may certainly be true. In this type of case, undergoing analysis is the answer.

PHYSICAL—Evidence in recent years suggests that, many times, it is an upset in the body chemistry that triggers a depressive state.

For instance, many other conditions manifest symptoms that mimic those of clinical depression, including *hypoglycemia* or *hyperglycemia* (blood sugar imbalance), high blood pressure, anemia, a thyroid or adrenal condition, and even diabetes. *All of these conditions are diet related.* They are successfully treated by correcting the dietary problem which caused them.

In other words, when nutrient-induced, the depressive state can be conquered by identifying the important element that is deficient (or in excess) in the body and then supplying (or removing) it. Although difficult to diagnose precisely, it's definitely not 'all in the mind' in many, many cases.

What we are stressing here is that very often a physical condition, *which can be identified by known diagnostic procedures,* is at the root of a depressive state. The important thing to understand is that hypoglycemia, hyperglycemia, a sluggish thyroid or exhausted adrenal gland can manifest themselves in extreme depression.

A six-hour glucose tolerance test is necessary to identify hypo (or hyper) glycemia; a simple blood test won't do it. A thyroid and/or adrenal gland that tests in the "average" normal range may not actually be functioning at a level high enough for that person's personal body chemistry. The "average" person just doesn't exist.

Before giving up and locking away a seriously depressed loved one, you simply must locate a very competent internist and diagnostician and (bully, browbeat, scream, holler) *insist* on a full range of tests to identify any possible physical cause.

TRYPTOPHAN—Although it requires competent medical advice and the proper prescription to correct it, depression has been traced to a chemical imbalance in the brain. This is a perfect example of the wonders just adding one simple supplement to the diet can bring. *Tryptophan* is an essential amino acid that the body requires to produce *serotonin.* Serotonin (a *neurotransmitter*) is necessary for efficient transmission of the electrical impulses that cause the brain and nerves to function. Science says that when tryptophan levels are low, leading to a deficiency in serotonin, behavior and personality are adversely affected.

In a landmark study, British medical researchers determined that supplying natural tryptophan to clinically depressed patients was just as effective as giving the antidepressant drug *imipramine.* All patients in the program recovered their spirits within four weeks, but the individuals on natural tryptophan suffered fewer side effects than those on the drug.

In another British study mounted to compare the value of

tryptophan versus the well-publicized 'shock treatment' (electro-convulsive shock treatment), the scientists reported that the results of the tryptophan treatment were superior to those of electric shock therapy. (In this experiment, the doctors used a daily supplement of 3 grams of tryptophan coupled with 1 gram of Vitamin B3 (niacinomide.) Studies conducted in Sweden, Norway, Denmark, and Finland confirm these findings.

Although tryptophan is present in many foods, including eggs, milk, cheese, and turkey, medical science says that just adding a high amount of these foods to the diet isn't the answer. Tryptophan is more readily effective in stimulating the production of serotonin when consumed as a supplement. (Note: Only a chemical analysis can identify a tryptophan deficiency. You *must* have competent medical advice.)

SAD - Seasonal Affective Disorder

LET THERE BE LIGHT—If you or someone you love goes into progressively worse depression during dark winter days, here's the explanation: The National Institute of Mental Health in Washington D.C. has confirmed the important findings of Dr. Norman Rosenthal of The Oregon Health Department, as follows:

SAD afflicts a relatively small proportion of persons (5 percent) living in areas of the country where gray winter skies keep people indoors. Dr. Rosenthal has determined that winter depression (related to the body's production of the hormone *melatonin*) is triggered by a lack of light, and it doesn't have to be sunlight either.

A simple cure for SAD is the use of a 3 foot by 4 foot box containing full-spectrum fluorescent tubing covered by a grid. (*Full-spectrum* light is the operative word here. Dr. Rosenthal uses Vita-Lite tubing. The cost of his box is $500 and it is available only by prescription. However, a handyman might be able to construct one at a much lower cost. The user is instructed never to look directly into the light box, just as we never look directly at the sun.)

Dr. Rosenthal instructs his patients to spend two or three hours daily in the presence of the light box. He reports that after using the light for just one week, depression lifts and the person becomes alert, happy, and feels alive again. During his study of this therapy, Dr. Rosenthal discovered that keeping a patient from the light for three weeks resulted in the renewed onset of the depressive state.

Note: The SAD syndrome can be inherited. If Junior is a happy, sunny youngster during summer, but becomes withdrawn and can't handle school during the winter months, he isn't necessarily learning-disabled. Give him a few hours per day in the presence of full-spectrum light and see what happens.

Overcoming Depression Naturally

If you feel that you, or a family member, may be slipping around the bend into a depressive state, the first step is a thorough physical examination and diagnostic tests to determine any organic or chemical imbalance in the system. You will, of course, follow doctor's orders in regard to any adjunctive tryptophan treatment or hormonal therapy for a low-functioning thyroid or or adrenal gland. You will, of course, modify your diet and make sure you are supplying optimum nutrients for efficent bodily functioning while eliminating any possible allergens targeted by your medical advisor. But there are several other areas of your life that you must examine as well.

REFUSING STRESS—During medieval times when the reigning King had the power of life and death, a robber was brought before a monarch known for his wicked delight in torturing prisoners to death. The trembling thief pleaded for his life most eloquently, but the King sentenced him to be drawn and quartered, a particularly nasty way to die. With a rush of adrenalin coursing through his system and certainly in the throes of extreme stress, the robber stuttered out a desperate proposition.

"Oh great and compassionate Monarch," he said. "Spare my life and I will dedicate my great talent to you. I will teach your steed to speak. 'Tis a secret I alone possess."

"Ridiculous!" thundered the King. "No one can teach a horse to talk."

"If I can't teach your beast to speak within one year, most great and terrible Majesty, then you can put me through the most unspeakable torture until I give up my mortal soul. Give me but one year to prove myself."

The King agreed and the thief was chained in the stall occupied by the monarch's favorite horse so that he would be near the beast but couldn't escape. The stableboys laughed and made great sport of him, but the robber laughed back and his happy disposition soon made him a favorite in the great stables. Finally one of the horse keepers asked him how he could be so happy in such adverse circumstances. He explained:

"Why should I not be merry? I cannot change my sad situation, but have I not persuaded the King to give me a year of life?"

"But what good will a year do ye, thief? Certainly you'll not tell me you can make that beast speak?"

"Ah, friend, you've missed the whole point. *Nothing is certain in this life but that circumstances will change.* I have a year. During that time the King may forget, or the King may die. I may die. Or, who knows? The horse *might* speak!"

STRESS—If your nerves are continually on edge because of stress (in your marriage, on the job, the kids, traffic, and so on), you must learn to simply refuse delivery of stress *if the situation itself is beyond your control.* It takes practice, but when you can't affect the *cause* of stress, you can refuse to allow it to affect you adversely.

If your boss is a real bear and you can't change jobs for one reason or another, learn to recognize and accept him for what he is. Really, who cares? Let his wife put up with him. He won't be a part of your life forever. If there's one thing certain in life, it's change. And, if the traffic is bumper-to-bumper and that road hog in front of you cuts in, so what? You can't control the traffic flow, so don't let it get to you. That's the whole point. If you can't control the situation, don't let the situation control you.

That anger coupled with temper which causes the adrenalin to rush into the bloodstream is nature's way of preparing us for *'fight or flight.'* But in our modern society, most of the time we don't run and we don't fight - and that's where we get into trouble. Learn to express your irritation. Get it over with and then let it go. You only hurt yourself by harboring feelings of revenge and anger. This leads to feelings of guilt which lead to depression because you're disappointed in yourself.

EXERCISE—Work it off! Punish your Rebounder (See *Rebounding,* Chapter 1), ride a bike, take a hike, go dancing, work up a healthy sweat on the tennis court or golf course. Do something physical and see how much better you feel.

RELAX—After a hard day at work, followed by a hard workout, let it all hang out and just relax. A good night's sleep "knits the raveled sleeve of care," as Shakespeare so aptly put it. You'll sleep soundly and awake refreshed if you have refused mental stress and stressed your body instead.

THINK POSITIVE—Every day in every way things are getting better and better. I'm OK and you're OK. This is the first day of the rest of your life. Believe and all things shall come unto you. If you don't fancy any of these popular sentiments, develop your own magic mantra.

MOTHER GOOSE—The Serenity prayer is beautifully phrased and certainly contains 'words to live by.' You might be surprised to learn that a little Mother Goose rhyme expresses the same thought. Here's how it goes:

> "For every evil under the sun,
> There be a remedy, or there be none.
> If there be one, seek till ye find it.
> If there be none, never mind it."

A Concluding thought

CONTROL—Stop trying! You can't control every facet of your life any more than anyone else can. It's trying to control everything around us that builds the stress which does us in. Go with the flow and laugh at adversity. The only thing really certain is change. Nothing lasts forever but the earth and sky. Even though you don't personally direct it, the sun *will* shine again on fertile green fields - and in your life.

CHAPTER 20

Chronic Insomnia

Natural Aids for Healthy Sleep

INSOMNIA—The last late movie is over and the last television station has signed off the air for the night. The entire household has been asleep for hours, but the chronic insomniac is wakeful and restless (and resentful). His bed linen is rumpled and tangled. His pillow has been pounded many times during the dark hours by his frustrated fists into what he hopes will be the magic shape.

He rises angrily and pads out to the kitchen where he raids the refrigerator, hoping to quiet his jangling nerves. He looks disgustedly out the window as he munches or wanders around the darkened house. He keeps an anxious eye on the clock because he has to go to work in a few hours. Finally he reaches into the medicine cabinet for one of the common over-the-counter sleep inducers. He's groggy for most of the following day from lack of sleep and the chemicals he ingested.

That night, determined not to go through the same search for sleep all over again, he takes sleep inducing drugs and retires early. Then, afraid that he won't sleep without drugs, he takes them nightly thereafter and unwittingly creates a chemical dependency in his system. All too soon, the pattern is set and his body *does* require the sleep-inducing chemicals. What was once an irrational fear has become truth.

Down through the ages, insomniacs desperate for sleep have tried everything from sipping hot milk to choking down several raw onions just before retiring to exercising themselves into a state of physical exhaustion. In today's drug-oriented society, it's much easier just to swallow a couple of pills. With sedatives, sleeping pills, and tranquilizers so easy to get, they can't be harmful - can they?

The Chemical Sleep-Inducers

A LOOK BACK—*Opium,* the great-great-grandfather of all sedatives, tranquilizers, anesthetics, and pain-killers, was listed in *De Materia Medica* by Dioscorides in the first century A.D. Assyrian cuneiform writing gave instruction on the extraction of opium (known as "lion fat") from the opium poppy. Prim and proper Victorian maidens and matrons alike took *laudanum,* a volatile mixture of alcohol and opium, for nervous 'vapors.' In fact, for many centuries, opium and alcohol were the only drugs available for use as sedatives, tranquilizers, anesthetics, or pain-relievers.

The first synthetic sedative, *chloral hydrate,* was introduced in 1869. This derivative of ethyl alcohol was warmly welcomed by a waiting public and its widespread use stimulated additional development of drugs with similar action. In the early 1900s, paraldehyde, amylene hydrate, sulfonmethan, and barbital were introduced. In 1912, phenobarbital arrived on the scene. During the next 20 years, a whole series of barbiturates were developed and even more types of sedative drugs were introduced in the 1950s. By the 1980s, over 150 different drugs with sedative properties had become available throughout the world. Without exceptions, each and every one of these drugs is highly addictive.

WE'VE COME A LONG WAY—To alleviate his night anxieties, all early man had to do was keep a fire burning at the mouth of his cave to keep wild beasts from attacking his family while all slept. The anxieties that keep the caveman's counterpart of today (male or female) from sleeping are far more complex.

In search of an immediate solution to the problem, we go

running to the doctor with our anxieties complaining of sleeplessness and come out clutching a prescription. Will it more surprise you to learn that only antibiotics are prescribed with more frequency than are sedatives and tranquilizers? Note: This chapter does not include a discussion of prescribed sleeping pills or tranquilizers. We will not presume to second-guess a knowledgeable and caring physician.

We are, however, taking a hard look at some of the more popular sleep-inducers that are readily available at the corner drug store. Sales of over-the-counter sleep aids are escalating yearly. In order not to lose a share of this lucrative market, more and more drug companies are putting out sleep-inducing products. Millions of dollars are spent on promotional advertising to convince the consumer of the merits of a particular brand.

Over-The-Counter Sleep Aids

WHAT'S IN A NAME?— Pardon us for not mentioning brand names, but the over-the-counter sleep-inducing products are almost interchangeable anyway. To test the truth of this statement, all you have to do is compare the active ingredient listed on each box. Although the product may contain a number of ingredients, most often only one single ingredient is listed as "active."

ANTIHISTAMINES—By far, the most common active ingredient used in over-the-counter sleep aids is an *antihistamine*, such as Doxylamine Succinate or Diphenhydramine HCL (hydrochloride). You know what an antihistamine is. You probably occasionally purchase cold or sinus remedies containing antihistamines to relieve the symptoms of those common maladies.

Unless these antihistamine-based cold and sinus relievers also contain caffeine (or a similar stimulant), the label carries the message that they can produce drowsiness. What is a potentially dangerous side-effect in medications designed to combat the common cold has been turned into a major feature of the over-the-counter sleep-inducing products. This has to be one of the real triumphs of manufacturing.

ACETAMINOPHEN—At least one of the major sleep-aids lists acetaminophen as its active ingredient. Just how this common pain reliever can turn into a sleep-inducing drug is a mystery. Perhaps the theory behind this product is the relief of minor body aches that can sometimes interfere with the normal process of drifting off to sleep.

Warning

ON THE LABEL—The usual warning on the labeling of over-the-counter sleep inducers cautions that the product should not be used by persons who have asthma, glaucoma, or an enlarged prostate, and should not be used for longer than two weeks. We are advised to consult a physician or a local Poison Control Center immediately in cases of an overdose.

OFF THE LABEL—Additional contraindications, (pertaining to antihistamines), not usually carried on the label itself, warn that these products should not be taken by a pregnant woman or nursing mother; that they should not be used by anyone with a peptic ulcer, a duodenal or bladder obstruction; that in the elderly (defined as over sixty years of age), they may cause dizziness and hypotension (low blood pressure). Diphenhydramine hydrochloride, in particular, must be used very cautiously (if at all) by persons with a history of cardiovascular disease, hypertension (high blood pressure), or a thyroid abnormality.

DANGEROUS SIDE-EFFECTS—Antihistamines can cause potentially dangerous side-effects in sensitive or susceptible persons (or with long-term use). In the *Nervous System:*

Dizziness, disturbed coordination, fatigue, confusion, restlessness, excitation, nervousness, tremors, irritability, blurred vision, tinnitus (noises in the ear), labyrinthitis (a condition of the inner ear resulting in loss of balance), hysteria, neuritis, and convulsions. In the *Cardiovascular System:* Heart palpitations, tachycardia (abnormally rapid heartbeat), hypotension (low blood pressure). In the *Gastrointestinal Tract:* Nausea, vomiting, diarrhea, constipation, anorexia, gastric distress. In the *Genito-Urinary System;* Suppressed urine, frequent urination, painful urination, early menses. In the *Respiratory System:* Nasal stuffiness, tightness of chest, wheezing, a thickening of the bronchial secretions. *General Adverse Reactions:* Anaphylactic shock, excessive perspiration, chills, dryness of mouth, nose, and throat, and skin rashes.

Admittedly, few of us suffer side-effects this severe. With occasional use, we have to assume the sleep-inducing drugs (whether prescribed or purchased over-the-counter) are safe when taken as directed. But let's examine the alternative of using natural sleep aids as a very pleasant contrast to flooding the body with chemicals.

The Natural Sleep Aids

THE NUTRIENTS—One of the problems with sleep-inducing drugs is that they tend to suppress dream episodes, evidenced by a lack of REM (rapid eye movement) sleep. Scientists are not sure just why REM sleep is so important. But when we sleep without dreaming, we have trouble concentrating during the next waking period. The subconscious appears to conjure up split-second fragments of undreamed dreams which interfere with mental focus. They come and go so fast that you probably are unaware of what's happening, but concentrating on the task at hand becomes difficult. Fortunately, some natural nutrients promote healthy normal sleep and allow you to wake refreshed (not groggy) the next day. Mother Nature takes care of her own.

Tryptophan: This natural amino acid is at the top of the nutrient list. As a rich source of tryptophan, milk really is a powerful sleep aid. When you sip that time-honored cup of milk at bedtime (warm or cold), you are supplying your body with the tryptophan it needs to manufacture *serotonin*. Serotonin is a neurotransmitter the brain requires for normal sleep.

In experiments conducted at the nation's research centers where sleep disorders are investigated, volunteers given tryptophan discovered that they fell asleep more quickly, enjoyed a longer period of time in deep sleep, and their sleep was uninterrupted. Monitoring of the subjects corroborated these facts.

If you tend to scoff at the sleep promoting effects of a cup of milk with its healthy content of tryptophan or have decided "it's all in the mind," you should know that animals can be sedated with tryptophan. It's certainly unlikely that an animal would be affected psychologically.

Bananas are another good food containing tryptophan, but milk remains the very best source. Please select the low-fat variety.

Calcium: Another reason why milk is such an excellent sleep aid is its content of *calcium*, often called "nature's tranquilizer." A continuing supply of calcium is needed to control sensory impulses, transmitted through the nerves. When the blood is low in calcium, the brain sends out a call for this mineral. A deficiency in calcium keeps you jumpy and unable to sleep until the body's requirement is satisfied. Low-fat dairy products, including that nightly cup of milk, will provide the calcium your body may be calling for. (A delicious sleeping potion highly favored abroad consists of stirring a tablespoon of raw honey into a cup of warm milk.) Additional food sources of calcium include raw seeds (sesame seeds are particularly good) and green leafy vegetables.

Arginine & Ornithine: One of the chemical changes which occurs in the brain and body during normal sleep is the release of *growth hormones* (GH). If the onset of sleep is delayed (or if the sleeping period is interrupted), the release of GH is delayed, interrupted, or eliminated altogether. Normal levels of GH play a vital part in keeping the immune system functioning efficiently.

(The elderly, in particular, often suffer from a lack of GH.)

Arginine and *ornithine* have been shown to increase the levels GH in the body. Chicken offers a relatively large supply of these two important amino acids and is the best food source. Southern fried chicken may be a toothsome delight, but the chicken parts absorb too much unhealthy fat when fried. Please roast or bake your chicken and don't eat the skin.

Choline & Lecithin: Both choline (an amine) and lecithin (a phospholipid (fat)) are precursors of *acetylcholine,* meaning that the body requires choline and/or lecithin to produce acetylcholine. Acetylcholine is a neurotransmitter used by the brain to regulate and control motion and sensory activities. (A deficiency of acetylcholine has been implicated in the onset of Alzheimer's disease). Bee pollen is an exceptionally rich food source of both choline and lecithin. Please see *Bee Pollen* (Chapter 13).

B Vitamins: Recent research indicates that *niacin* (B3) acts as one of the natural neurotransmitters which affects sleep, explaining why people who take large doses of niacin find that they are sleepy, but typically have difficulty falling asleep.

B12 is another safe sleep promoting part of B-complex. Unless you already take a healthy dose of B-complex every day, B12 has a very interesting side-effect. When 1,000 micrograms of B12 are taken *immediately* before retiring, the colors occuring in dreams are vividly enhanced. The body rapidly builds a tolerance to this effect and it soon disappears. But those who have experienced it say it is really spectacular!

Brewer's yeast supplies a goodly amount of the B vitamins that promote sleep. The experts say that taking two heaping tablespoons of brewer's yeast at bedtime (in a cup of warm broth) will guarantee a good night's rest. Other food sources of the Bs include organ meats, wheat germ, bran, whole grains, and green vegetables. Mushrooms are a particularly good source of niacin.

Note: Taking a large dose of niacin (converted to *niacinamide* by the body) usually results in what is termed "the niacin flush." The entire body flushes red and feels very warm. Many also complain of an uncontrollable itching sensation after a dose of niacin. This is a temporary condition and is not harmful, but the flush and itching can last for several uncomfortable hours. And, if your're not expecting the niacin flush, these sensations can be frightening. Another form of B3, *nicotinamide,* produces only a mild flush and may be preferred by those sensitive to niacin or niacinamide.

THE BOTANICALS—The modern medical doctor and the pharmacist he relies upon to dispense the pills and liquids manufactured in giant laboratories owe a lot more to the early herbalists than they might think. It was not until the end of the 19th century, the relatively recent past when you consider mankind's long history, that the secrets of preparing synthetic drugs and medicines began to be discovered. It is a fact that the active elements of many plants remain the basis for a surprising number of today's drugs. But long before science learned how to synthesize chemical drugs, the healers of antiquity were working miracles with the medicinal botanicals.

Chamonile—Chamomile (*Matricaria chamomilla*) is one of the oldest and most important of the medicinal herbs. In fact, Chamomile was so highly regarded by ancient Egyptian physicians, it was dedicated to their highest diety, the Sun God. In the Middle Ages, sweet-smelling and fragrant Chamomile was always included in the fresh straw and herbs strewn on dank castle floors to sweeten the air and cushion the feet from the rough stones, as well as being one of the premiere herbs in the medicine bag.

Herbalists say that Chamomile is a powerful sleep inducer. It soothes jangled nerves, calms the stomach, and woos slumber. In the mid-1970s, two New York cardiologists decided to test the effects of Chamomile tea on twelve heart patients who were scheduled for cardiac catheterization. (This very painful procedure consists of introducing a catheter directly into the heart through an arm vein.) All of the patients were understandably anxious and dreading undergoing the catheterization, but agreed to take a cup of Chamomile tea beforehand.

The physicians were amazed to find that ten of their patients actually fell asleep during the procedure itself! The doctors explained, "It is most unusual for patients undergoing cardiac catheterization to fall asleep. The anxiety produced by this procedure as well as the pain associated with cardiac catheterization all but preclude the ability to sleep. Further investigation of the role of Chamomile tea as a sedative is warranted."

If Chamomile can induce sleep during a painful medical procedure, certainly conquering insomnia must be child's play for this ancient and powerful herb. To guarantee swift slumber, don't rely on Chamomile teabags. Purchase only whole dried flowers. Pour 6 ounces of freshly boiled water over six or eight of the florets, cover, and steep for five minutes. Strain off the herb residue, sweeten to taste with raw honey, if you like. Sip warm about a half an hour before retiring.

Hops—Hops (Humulus Lupulus) is best known as an important ingredient in beer brewing where it imparts the characteristic bitter taste. It is the content of volatile oils in Hops which produce a sedative and soporific effect. Hops both improve the appetite and promote sleep. An old herbal says that Hops is "much given in nervousness and hysteria and at bedtime to induce sleep, frequently procuring sleep for the patient after long periods of sleeplessness in overwrought conditions of the brain."

Hops botanical name *Humulus* is believed to have originated from the fact that Hops prefer a rich, moist humus as its growing medium. *Lupulus* may have come the Latin term for wolf (lupus). The Roman naturalist, Pliny the Elder (A.D. 23-79), tells us that when grown among other plants, Hops "strangles them by its light, climbing embraces, as the wolf does a sheep." Hops English name comes from the Anglo-Saxon term *hoppan* (to climb).

Fresh Hops flowers and leaves, the medicinal part of the herb, have a strong odor and very bitter taste. Only very recently dried Hops (still greenish in color) can be used because the odor and taste becomes very unpleasant the longer they are kept. To brew an infusion (tea) of Hops as a bedtime sleep aid, pour 6 ounces of freshly boiled water over a rounded tablespoon of the fresh herb parts, cover, and steep for five minutes. Strain off the residue, and sip while warm about a half an hour before retiring. It is best not to sweeten this tea.

If you want to prepare a *tincture* of Hops, an old recipe directs that you loosely fill a glass bottle (not plastic) with the flowers and a few leaves. Add enough pure "spirits" (vodka will do nicely) to cover the herb parts. Cork, and allow the bottle to remain undisturbed in a warm place for about two weeks. Take a small "wineglass" full before going to bed. In herbal lore, a "wineglass" equates to a scant two ounces.

Valerian—Valerian (*Valeriana officinalis*) was so highly esteemed in medieval times that it was known as "All Heal." Most authorities believe its name comes from the Latin *valere,* meaning "to be in health." There are over 150 varieties of this potent botanical and references to Valerian's medicinal properties date back to Biblical times, The Spikenard mentioned in the Bible as being used to anoint Jesus Christ was an aromatic ointment that many authorities believe was produced from one of the members of the Valerian family.

A quite remarkable use for Valerian as detailed in 14th century writings directs: "Men who begin to fight and when you wish to stop them, give to them the juice of Valeriana and peace will be made immediately." This rather startling little bit of history is undoubtedly a comment on the sedative and tranquilizing qualities of this herb.

An early herbal says "Valerian allays pain and promotes sleep. It is of especial use and benefit to those suffering from nervous overstrain as it possesses none of the after-effects produced by narcotics." The juice of the fresh root, sold under the name *Energetene of Valerian* in Britain (where Valerian is still commerically grown), is recommended as a powerful sleep aid for the insomniac.

The rhizome (root) of Valerian is where the herb stores its

medicinal properties. The dried root of this herb may be purchased. Because the true Valerian root is often mixed with lesser species, follow the package directions to brew your slumber inducing infusion. *Note:* Used in small amounts, Valerian is wonderfully quieting and soothing to the brain and nervous system, but this very powerful and potent herb must be treated with respect. Large doses, if repeated too frequently, may result in a headache, a feeling of heaviness, apathy, or stupor

The Herb Pillow—Although the origin of this sleep promoting use of herbs is lost in antiquity, many of the sweet-scented herbs have been used to freshen stagnant room air and stale garments since time immemorial. First used only in their short-lived fresh form, clever fingers probably discovered early on that they could fashion sachets by stitching bits of the dried herbs into tiny plump pillows. From tiny sachets to bed pillows was the logical next step.

The most pleasant way I know of to waft off to sleep is by tucking an herb pillow under your heavy head. The use of herbs in external poultices for various conditions undoubtedly led to the discovery that breathing in the scent of certain dried herbs exerts the most remarkable soporific effect. Recent research coming out of central Europe and the U.S.S.R. confirms that premise. It appears that when the heat of the body gently warms a specific blending of dried herbs, breathing in the vapors thus released promotes a deep healthy sleep.

Although these special sleep promoting herbs pillows are easy to find abroad, they are sometimes difficult to locate "ready-made" in the U.S. If you decide to try your hand at making one, you will need a quantity of dried: Anise, Bee Balm (or Lemon Balm), Chamomile, Hops, Lavender, Peppermint, Rosemary, Sage, Thyme (common), and Thyme (wild).

Begin by blending equal parts of each herb. Then add additional Hops balanced by extra handfuls of Lavender and Peppermint until you have achieved a pleasing scent. Using very tightly woven cloth (so that the herbs parts cannot poke through and disturb an unwary sleeper), cut two squares. Stitch three sides of your pillow together using a small gauge stitch. Fill loosely with the herb blend and stitch the fourth side closed.

If this sounds like too much trouble, or if you're not a seamstress, you'll be happy to know that we have located a mail-order source of these sleep promoting herb pillows in the U.S. This company carries many hard-to-find health related items and will be happy to send you a catalog on request. Contact *New Dimensions Distributors,* 2419 N. Black Canyon Highway, Suite 7, Phoenix, Arizona 85009. Call 1-800-624-7114 toll-free.

Note: If you're interested in taking a fascinating look at the way herbs have been used through past centuries and into modern times, *Miracle Healing Power Through Nature's Pharmacy* (Fisher Publishing, Canfield, Ohio) is both a practical guide (with 32 full-color plates) to the use of the medicinal botanicals and is most entertaining as well.

"White Noise"

NIGHT NOISES—No matter how familiar you are with the creaks and groans that your house makes in the night, very often you find yourself wide awake and monitoring these night noises when you should be sleeping. (Oh, the refrigerator just clicked on. That's the furnace rumbling, did I forget to turn down the thermostat? I must remember to trim the tree; that darn tree branch is scraping at the window again. The wind is whistling down the chimney; it must be going to rain.)

WHITE NOISE—A "white" noise is a monotonous rhythmic sound that often has an almost hypnotic effect on the insomniac. You might try the hum of a fan, the steady tick-tock of a wind-up clock, or some barely discernible soft music playing on your bedside radio. (The bedtime lullaby still works.) Some manufacturers are even marketing white noise devices that make it easy to go to sleep. Originally designed to assist daytime sleepers who work the nightshift, these machines have proven valuable to insomniacs as well.

Before investing cold cash in a manufactured device, you might want to try one of the suggestions given above first. Research says that a white noise can lull the most hard-core insomniac quickly to sleep.

Practice Sleeping

Many respected authorities believe we can train the body to go to sleep, just as we can train the body to perform other tasks. The recommended method is to take two daily practice sessions of at least thirty minutes each. You may want to give your body a few lessons. Here's how:

In a darkened room, comfortably lie down on your back and allow your body to go completely limp. Beginning with your toes and working upwards, tense each group of muscles and hold tight for a count of ten. Relax and allow the tension to dissipate before proceeding to the next area of the body. Alternately tense and relax each separate group of muscles (up to and including the neck, face, and even the eyes) before continuing.

Make a conscious effort to feel the tension draining away from each group of muscles as you proceed. The idea is to help your body learn to differentiate between muscles held unconsciously tense and muscles consciously loose and relaxed. On top of your practice sessions, use this method to completely relax at bedtime also. The experts say that once this technique has been learned, sleep comes swiftly on the heels of released tension.

Happy Dreams

There are documented cases of certain rare individuals who appear to live and work efficiently on very little sleep. Some of these persons, like Einstein and Edison, were accustomed to frequent cat naps. Others just plain don't require the proverbial eight hours of sleep every night. If you are stuck on the notion that eight hours of sleep is an iron-clad requirement, try going to bed an hour or so later than your normal bedtime and see if you fall asleep more easily. Relax beforehand with a cup of hot herb tea (or milk) and remember that your bed is a snug and welcome haven, not some medieval torture device. May the sandman visit you promptly and may all your dreams be sweet.

SURPRISE BONUS

The Dr. Steichen Sink & Strut

A Safe & Fun Little Exercise

In March of 1986, Fischer Publishing received a most delightful letter from Edward F. Steichen, M.D. of Lenora, Kansas. Dr. Steichen invited us to take a look at his "Universal Steichen's Safety Swinging Sink & Strut Exercise." Having read and approved the original *Hidden Secrets of Super-Perfect Health,* the doctor offered to allow us to incorporate the Sink & Strut in our writings. Dr. Steichen says his exercise regimen will "revitalize and energize you and give you a new long-term lease on life!" We agree.

Dr. Steichen was born in Tipton, Kansas on January 29, 1905. He worked on the family farm until he earned his A.B. degree from Kansas University, then entered medical school and received his M.D. from the University of Chicago in 1931. Dr. Steichen's dedicated service as a Family Practitioner was acknowledged by Governor Docking with a state proclaimed "Dr. Steichen Day" commemorating his more than 40 years of both community service and doctoring. This beloved doctor was honored state-wide with a program and parade that was covered and televised by A.B.C.

This dynamo served the State of Kansas for eight years in the House of Representatives. On top of his very busy medical practice, Dr. Steichen's past community involvement includes services on the School Board, in the City Council and as President of the Chamber of Commerce, and he also served as mayor of Lenora for six years. In fact, Dr. Steichen has had a hand in so many other areas of service to his community and state that it's impossible to list them all here. Suffice it to say that Dr. Steichen, now 81 years old, is a most remarkable man indeed. Mrs. Steichen (deceased) was a registered nurse and the couple had two sons, one daughter, and Dr. Steichen now boasts of eleven grandchildren!

As a result of a debilitating illness he suffered in 1976 which left him with severely weakened legs and precarious balance, Dr. Steichen developed the exercise program he credits with keeping him ambulatory. He says that this regimen is his "simple, *no cost,* world-wide answer to 'physical fitness,' available to any person who can stand up, even if they have to hold on."

We are very happy to recommend the "Steichen Sink & Strut" to one and all. Besides, it's fun! The entire staff of Fischer Publishing is swinging with the Strut and lovin' every minute of it.

The Steichen Sink & Strut

WHAT YOU NEED—You need a wrist-height horizontal support to grip onto and you already have all the "equipment" you need. Try out your bathroom sink, utility sink, kitchen sink, desk, foot of your bed, or porch railing to find out which is most comfortable for you. Kick any loose rugs out of the way to make sure your shoes won't slip. Put a chair beside you so that you can sit down and rest if you need to.

HERE'S HOW—Get and keep a firm grip on the horizontal support you have selected. Keep your elbows well bent at all times to maintain alternating muscle tension on arms, shoulders, and back through every movement of these exercises. This is your upper body workout as well as your leg and torso exercises. It can be done regardless of the weather, at any time of the day or night.

EXERCISE #1—Grip the support, bend your knees slightly, then slowly trot backwards while swinging your hips. Push against the support with your upper body muscles. Allow first your toes and then your heels to strike the floor with each step, remember to swing those hips from side to side! After you have trotted backwards while *pushing* as far as you can (and extended your body as close to horizontal as possible) for several minutes, gradually trot forward until you are *pulling* on your support with increasing force for several minutes. Dr. Steichen says it's easy to keep track if you count up to 100 steps as your right foot strikes, first while *pushing* and then while *pulling*. Remember to *keep your arms well bent at all times*. Then rise to an upright position while continuing to trot slowly. Rest for moment. Use the chair beside you if you need it - that's why it's there.

EXERCISE #2—In an upright position, place both feet two feet back (comfortably apart) while gripping firmly onto your horizontal support. You will be leaning forward slightly. Now bend at the knees and slowly allow your body to sink down as close to the floor as possible, then rise upright. Use your horizontal support to alternately push against and pull yourself up if need be. Repeat. Dr. Steichen says to *slowly* increase repeats until you can comfortably handle 25 times per session. Easy does it.

EXERCISE #3—Beginning in a standing position while keeping a firm grip on your horizontal support, bend at the knees and slowly allow your body to sink down backwards until your buttocks almost touch your heels, then spring upwards. Try to *extend your jump* by using your arms and hands to push yourself as high as possible. Repeat as many times as comfortable. Dr. Steichen recommends you slowly work up to 25 times per session.

EXERCISE #4—While maintaining a firm grip on your horizontal support, allow your head to turn first to the right, then left, then drop forward, then backward. This exercise will help limber up your neck muscles and joints. Continue the movements in sequence for a few moments, but beware of dizziness.

Dr. Steichen Says:

"Remember, you should consult with your physician before starting any exercise program. These exercises can be done a few minutes or more at a time several times a day, or more times all at once - whatever your physical condition or busy schedule will allow. If you become tired after a few minutes, take several deep breaths and get your second wind before continuing."

"MONITOR YOUR PULSE RATE—As soon as you complete my Sink & Strut routine, sit down on the chair you have ready beside you and count your pulse. A rate of 120 to 130 is considered safe for most people doing these exercises but check with your physician.

If you find it difficult to check your own pulse, try this: Turn your right hand palm up. Using just the tips of the first and second fingers of your left hand, press lightly but firmly just to the right of the ligaments that run down the center of your right wrist. This is the radial artery and you should feel the blood pulsing through it quite easily.

You can count beats for 15 seconds and multiply by four, but counting beats for 30 seconds (or even a full 60 seconds) is much more accurate."

"EXERCISE YOUR "WILL" POWER—It won't cost you a penny to replace *won't power* with *will power*! You'll progress far beyond your second childhood at no cost but will power. You too can face the world in your personal best physical condition when you use my Sink & Strut."

When done properly, these exercises will exert every muscle in your body (from fingers to toes) to their fullest extent by pushing, pulling, jumping, twisting, and grasping *safely*. Do these exercises (or part of them) just one to three minutes several times or more daily for a month or two as a beginner until you can work into a regular routine which lasts 20 to 30 minutes. After you have the routine down pat, turn on some music and sink and strut to your favorite beat!"

Aches & Pains

LATE-BREAKING NEWS—A warming all-natural massage creme being sold in the US. under the trademarked name of *Medicreme*™ may be of particular interest to you. This creme was discovered on our last fact-finding tour of Europe, where it is used with great benefit by those suffering from arthritis, bursitis, rheumatism, and chronic back pain, as well as by champion athletes.

In additon to its long history of successful use in Europe, Medicreme™ has been field-tested extensively by John Orsini, a former member of the U.S.A. championship Olympic weight-lifting team, and carries his personal endorsement. You may know John Orsini better as the President of All-American Health & Fitness and the developer of All-American Sports Vitamins. Mr. Orsini says nothing beats Medicreme™ for sore, aching muscles (no matter what the cause) and pulled, overworked or strained muscles. This original European formula creme generates a penetrating heat that soothes and heals aches and pains with its all-natural secret herbal ingredients. You'll know it's working by the healthy warm flush of your skin as it penetrates to increase blood circulation in the area. New to the U.S., Medicreme™ is not yet in wide distribution, but top health food stores should carry it soon. For mail order service, please see the following chapter for ordering information.

EPILOGUE

Now Is The Time

Today is the First Day of the Rest of Your Life

Both individuals and families all around the world have begun demanding that the information they need to preserve or regain their good health be made available to them. The doctor isn't perceived as a god anymore and the pronouncements of medical science are no longer being received as proclamations from Mt. Olympus. We are in a questioning phase. We are asking hard questions and we are demanding substantial answers.

What We Don't Know Can Hurt Us

Self-Care Health-Care is the order of the day. We're just not happy with the way the 'experts' have taken care of us. The health of the nation is threatened by polluted soils and polluted waters. We are not pleased to find that commercial interests dictate the way our foods are supplied to us. We are not content to continue heedlessly traveling down the old roads that led to the so-called 'diseases of civilization,' including heart disease and cancer, that threaten society today. The only solution is to gain enough knowledge so that we can protect ourselves. *Hidden Secrets of Super-Perfect Health, Book II,* is our contribution to the growing body of knowledge on effective preventive medicine that you told us you want and need.

For Your Convenience

Although most of the products discussed in *Hidden Secrets, Book II*, are available in major health food stores nationwide, you may sometimes have trouble locating a particular item that seems just right for you.

When that time comes, or if you just plain prefer arm-chair shopping convenience, we suggest you request a catalog from *New Dimensions Distributors*. This forward-thinking organization carries many hard-to-find health-related products and devices. You'll like the friendly staff, toll-free ordering, prompt service, and their selection of quality products. Here's their address:

New Dimensions Distributors
2419 N. Black Canyon Highway, Suite #7
Phoenix, Arizona 85009
Call Toll-Free 1-800-624-7114 - Extension 18
In Arizona Call: (602) 257-1183

Take The First Step

The longest journey in the world begins with but a single step. We can bring you the health care information you need to protect yourself, but we can't undertake the journey for you. Only you can put the knowledge gleaned from our many, many years of study and research into practice so that it works for you. Armed with old and new knowledge presented within these pages, take that all-important first step *now*.

INDEX

A
acetaminophen - 261
acne - 130, 185
acupressure - 90
acupuncture - 90
adenosine - 59
adrenalin - 256
aerobic exercise - 14, 16
alfalfa - 66, 230, 246, 247
allicin - 57, 59, 60, 63, 65
almonds - 142, 206, 207, 214
amygdalin - 206, 207, 214
androgen - 133
anemia - 251
angina - 7, 68, 126, 225, 226, 227, 228, 229, 242
antibiotics - 62, 169
antihistamines - 260-261
appendicitis - 104, 110
arginine - 263-264
arteriosclerosis - 58, 70, 75, 126, 154
arthritis - 4, 7, 28, 34, 75, 126, 229, 230, 240, 241, 245, 247
Aspartame (see NutraSweet)
asthma - 58, 126, 128
atherosclerosis - 43, 59, 60, 68, 77, 78, 83, 126, 154, 225, 226, 227, 228, 231, 232
athletes - 169-170
atonic colon - 108
auriculotherapy - 91

B
backaches - 5
Banting, Sir Frederick - 44
barbiturates - 259
bee pollen - 91, 140-141, 149-155, 158, 160, 166-174, 264
beta-carotene - 27, 28, 211
bile - 107
bioflavonoids (See Vitamin P)
Bio-Strath - 174-177
birth control pills - 89
blood clots - 58

blood pressure - 33, 35, 58, 63, 78, 79, 82-83, 126, 150, 151, 152, 153, 154, 229, 241
blood type A - 216-217
bonemeal - 236, 246
botulism - 49
bowel obstruction - 109
bran - 246
Brewer's yeast - 99, 122, 233, 246, 264
bromelaine - 99, 215
bronchial problems - 58
Budwig, Dr. Johanna - 68-86
Burk, Dean - 200
bursitis - 4, 229

C
calcium - 152, 236, 263
cancer - 5, 28, 39, 43, 60-62, 70, 71, 72, 75, 81, 82, 104, 109, 116, 134-135, 136-137, 145, 169, 198-199, 200-201, 204-221
Candida utilis - 174-175, 177
capsicum - 66
carbohydrates - 39, 43, 44, 47, 50
carrot - 25-30
Carter, Al - 1, 7, 8, 9
castor oil - 113
cavities - 197-198
cayenne (See capsicum)
cesium - 214
Chamomile - 265-266
chloral hydrate - 259
cholesterol - 6, 39, 59, 126, 154, 225, 229, 231, 233, 237, 242, 243, 245
choline - 108, 119, 233, 234, 264
circulatory system - 32, 33, 36, 58, 89, 95, 124, 126, 130, 180, 242
clinical depression - 250
colitis - 43, 110, 114
collagen - 32, 188
common cold - 33, 34, 53, 64, 126
consensual reaction - 125

279

INDEX

constipation - 43, 89, 96, 99, 102, 103-123
cottage cheese - 68, 69

D

damiana - 146
Dastre-Moratsche (See consensual reaction)
depression - 44, 249-257
dermis - 187
DHEA - 213
diabetes - 32, 35, 40, 42, 43, 44, 64, 154, 251
diverticulitis - 43, 104, 110-111
diverticulosis - 104, 110
Dr. Rinse Formula - 222, 229-231, 233-248
Dr. Steichen Sink & Strut - 273-276
Dry-Brush Massage - 100, 178-184

E

eczema - 75, 94, 126
elastin - 188
ELF - 219, 220
epidermis - 187
Erickson, Dr. Eric H. - 166
eyesight - 17, 26, 119, 126, 245

F

Feverfew - 92
fiber - 99, 103, 104, 105
flax (See linseed oil)
flaxseed - 121, 122
fluoride - 193-203
F-M Circulizer System - 124-131, 154
food allergies - 88
footbath (See F-M Circulizer System)
frei öl - 189-192
full spectrum light - 253

G

garlic - 51-67, 100, 226
Garlic-Rose Elixir - 55

gastro-intestinal tract - 27, 75, 169
geopathogenic zones - 218-219
ginseng - 146, 172, 173
glucose - 39
Gotu kola - 172, 173-174
gout - 28
gravity - 9, 10
Groff, Laverne - 2-3

H

hair dryer - 91
Ha-ras gene - 217-218
headaches - 5, 43, 87-93, 250
heart disease - 39, 43, 58, 66, 68, 70, 71, 75, 77, 127, 145, 160, 224-225
heart rate - 15, 75, 126, 226, 275
hemorrhoids - 33, 43, 104, 109, 116
herbs - 91, 92, 100, 124, 125, 130, 268
honey - 47-49, 55, 92
hops - 266-267
hormones - 89
hydrogenation - 65
hyperglycemia - 251, 252
hypoglycemia - 42, 89, 241, 251, 252

I

immune system - 32, 75
impotence - 148-157
influenza - 33, 34, 126
inositol - 119, 234
insomnia - 126, 251, 258-271

J

Johnson, Noel - 149, 158-165

K

kelp - 246
kidneys - 126, 180
Kramb, Hanne - 145, 155-157

L

labyrinthitis - 34
lactic acid - 118
Laetrile - 205-208, 214

INDEX

Lancet - 45
laudanum - 259
laxatives - 112-115
lecithin - 100, 142, 226, 227, 232, 233, 244, 246, 264
Lind, Dr. James - 31
linoleate - 232
linseed oil - 28, 68-86, 142, 152, 155
lipoproteins - 232
liver - 58, 75, 97, 180
loofah - 182
lungs - 28, 75, 204
lymphatic system - 7, 11, 16

M

magnesium - 226, 235-236
manic-depression - 250
Medicreme - 276
Mendelsohn, Dr. Robert S. - 176
migraine (See headaches)
milk - 263
milk of magnesia - 114
mineral oil - 113
minerals - 27, 46, 58, 66, 108, 113, 114, 150, 166, 175
Miracles of Rebound Exercise, The - 9, 21, 24
miscarriage - 34
molasses - 46
monosodium glutamate - 88
multiple sclerosis - 75
muscles - 12-13
mustard seeds - 121, 122

N

NASA - 20, 158
natural bristle brush - 182
Nelson, Harris - 6-7
niacin - 119, 264
Nieper, Hans, M.D. - 208-209
nitrates - 88
nitrites - 88
Nixon, Richard - 204
NutraSweet - 45, 46, 49

O

oncogenes - 217
opium - 259
ornithine - 263
Orsini, John - 276
osteoporosis - 126, 227, 228, 247
ovarian problems - 2
overweight - 43, 84, 105, 151, 152, 210, 250

P

parsley - 53
penile prostheses - 139-140
peristalsis - 116, 121, 123
phenobarbital - 259
phenylalanine (See NutraSweet)
phlebitis - 94, 229
potassium - 107, 108, 120, 153
pregnancy - 79, 97
prostaglandins - 75-79
prostate - 75, 116, 126, 133-147
prostatectomy - 137-139
prostatic hypertrophy - 135-136
prostatitis - 135, 141, 169
psyllium - 121, 122
pumpkin seeds - 142

R

Reagan, Ronald - 159, 167
Rebound, The - 1, 22
rebound constipation - 114
Rebound Dynamics - 1, 20
rebounding - 1-24, 155, 256
rectal exam - 137
REM - 262
rheumatism - 28, 126, 247
Rinse, Jacobus, Ph. D. - 222-227
rose hips - 35
Rosemary - 92
Rosenthal, Norman, M.D. - 253
Ross, Walt & Dorothy - 4-6
royal jelly - 172-173
rubidium - 214

281

INDEX

S
saccharine - 43
SAD - 250, 253-254
Safe Water Foundation - 200
safflower oil - 226, 227, 244
salt - 151, 212
sandalwood - 184
scurvy - 31, 54
sebaceous glands - 185, 186, 187
sedatives - 259, 260
selenium - 211
semen - 133
serotonin - 252, 263
sexual function - 55, 71, 139
sharks - 213
sheep lice - 215-216
sinusitis - 127-128
skin 130, 179-184, 185-192
sleep aids - 259-271
Small Flowered Willow Herb - 143-145
Smith, Dr. Lendon H. - 176-177
smoking - 129, 151, 152, 154, 204, 225
sperm - 134
squalene - 213
staphylococcus infection - 80
Steichen, Dr. Edward F. - 272-273
sterility - 27
steroids - 215
Strathmeyer, Dr. Walther - 174
stress - 151, 153, 225, 254-255
sucrose - 39, 50
sugar (refined, white) - 37-50
sugar addiction - 40-42
sunflower seeds - 233, 246
support stockings - 100
Szent-Gyorgyi, Dr. Albert - 31

T
Testes - 133
thiamin - 120
thrombophlebitis - 94
tranquilizers - 260
tryptophan - 252-253, 262-263

U
ulcers - 29, 34, 43, 75
urea - 214
urethra - 133
U.S.S.R. - 63, 167, 268

V
Valerian - 267-268
varicose veins - 33, 43, 94-101, 109, 126, 245
Vervain - 92
Vinaigre des Quatre Voleurs - 57
Vitamin B Complex - 100, 104, 233, 234, 235, 264
Vitamin C - 31-36, 100, 226, 237, 246
vitamin deficiency - 28
Vitamin E - 97, 100, 108, 143, 191, 226, 238, 246
Vitamin P - 31-36, 99, 153, 155
vitamins - 27, 46, 58, 66, 107, 108, 113, 114, 150, 166, 175

W
wheat germ - 101, 120, 122, 142, 233, 246
whey - 118, 122
white noise - 269
wounds - 48

Y
yeast - 119
yeast infections - 58, 62
Yiamouyiannis, John, Ph.D. - 200

Z
zinc - 101, 141, 142, 216, 239, 246

Other Outstanding Books on Health And Natural Healing From Fischer Publishing

How To Survive In The Hospital by Joan Haas-Unger, RN
There are too many procedures, performed by too many doctors, in too many places, with too high a stroke-and-death rate. This landmark book can help you lower your risks and increase your chances of survival in the hospital.

ISBN 0-915421-06-2 $12.95

How To Fight Cancer And Win by William L. Fischer
It clearly spells out real cancer preventives and cures, many never before published, with strong scientific documentation and stories of miraculous cures. They are all presented in a concise easy-to-understand style. You can put this vast knowledge into practice to insure that this deadly disease never strikes home.

ISBN 0-915421-07-0 $14.95

The Miracle Healing Power Through Nature's Pharmacy by William L. Fischer
Now you can learn how to treat virtually every disease or condition known to man—naturally! A comprehensive guide to help you and heal you . . . the most complete . . . most useful . . . and most up to date work of its kind. Complete with many documented case histories and 32 full-color illustrations.

ISBN 0-915421-04-6 $19.95

fischer publishing   one fischer square   box 368   canfield, ohio 44406